Key Business Skills
for Nurse Managers

KEY BUSINESS SKILLS FOR NURSE MANAGERS

Leann Strasen, R.N., M.B.A.

Vice President, Henry Mayo Newhall Memorial Hospital
Valencia, California

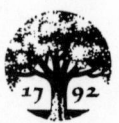

Philadelphia **J. B. LIPPINCOTT COMPANY**

London   New York   São Paulo   Mexico City   St. Louis   Sydney

Sponsoring Editor: Paul Hill
Manuscript Editor: Helen Ewan
Indexer: Barbara Littlewood
Art Director: Tracy Baldwin
Designer: Earl Gerhart

Production Manager: Kathleen P. Dunn
Production Coordinator: Carol A. Florence
Compositor: Digitype
Printer/Binder: R. R. Donnelley & Sons
Company

654321

Library of Congress Cataloging-in-Publication Data

Strasen, Leann
    Key business skills for nurse managers.

    Includes bibliographies and index.
    1. Nursing — Practice.   2. Business.   3. Nursing
service administration.   I. Title.   [DNLM: 1. Administrative
Personnel — education — nurses' instruction.
WY 18.5.S897b]
RT86.7.S77   1987   362.1'73'068   86-10699
ISBN 0-397-54574-6

Preface

KEY BUSINESS SKILLS for Nurse Managers was written to equip nurse managers and administrators with the business skills required to function effectively in the rapidly changing health care environment of the 1980s. Deregulation and increased competition in the health care industry have significantly changed the role and responsibilities of nursing managers in acute care institutions. As a result of these changes in responsibilities, additional skills and expertise in areas such as financial management, marketing, economics, strategic planning, and budgeting are needed for the nurse manager to be competitive and effective in the workplace.

Traditionally, nurses promoted to management positions were excellent clinical nurses having leadership potential and few skills or training in business disciplines. They received most of their indoctrination to specific management theories and skills as a result of on-the-job training.

This method of educating nurse managers is no longer adequate in the rapidly changing environment of health care delivery. The competitive health care workplace calls for the acquisition of skills and knowledge not traditionally included in any baccalaureate or master's program in nursing.

This textbook was developed for use in graduate programs in nursing administration and by the practicing nurse manager and administrator. There are no current textbooks that include the perspectives of the disciplines of economics, marketing, strategic planning, networking, budgeting, and financial applications for the nurse manager. The specific focus of this text is on the acute care institution because of the overwhelming demand for nursing management skills in this environment.

Key Business Skills for Nurse Managers was also written to assist the practicing nurse manager to expand his or her knowledge base to include specific skills from the business sector, such as budgeting, financial management, marketing, and cost accounting. It was designed to be easily read, understood, and applied by the practicing nurse manager/administrator.

The text was written to include for each of the areas a level of detail and depth that can be used on a daily basis by the manager. The text was not intended to provide the student with an in-depth knowledge of all of these disciplines, but rather to provide a generalist approach to business skills for the nurse manager. Entire books have been written on each individual topic in the text. The manager who has a strong interest in or need to gain additional expertise in a specific field is directed to in-depth texts on the specific topic.

The uniqueness of the text lies in the fact that an overview of major business skills is included in the same text with examples and applications specific to the nurse manager/administrator's daily operating environment. The examples and case studies presented include everyday situations which a nurse manager deals with on an ongoing basis.

The final two chapters, Networking Skills and Power and Politics in Health Care, are not topics traditionally included in a business school curriculum. It was felt, however, that these two areas are very important for and applicable to the potential success of the nurse manager in the current and future competitive health care environment. These skills are important and of interest to both the new and the experienced manager. For the new manager, the topics provide an overview of personal skills that are beneficial for a manager to acquire. For the experienced manager, these chapters may provide an explanation of why certain strategies have worked for them whereas others have not. They can provide a validation for various hypotheses the manager may have identified through his or her experience.

This text is a first attempt to consolidate information on business skills for the nurse manager. As the health care industry continues to become more like the private sector, many additional and in-depth texts on these topics will be required for nursing. As nurse managers acquire an understanding of these basic skills and terminology, their questions and inquiries will determine the texts that follow.

Leann Strasen, R.N., M.B.A.

Acknowledgments

SPECIAL THANKS are due to a number of professional colleagues who have been motivating forces throughout my educational and professional experience.

Those special thanks go to:

Charlotte Katona and Eula Das, my first two mentors, who displayed confidence in my abilities and encouraged me in my endeavors.

Duffy Watson, for his inspirational leadership over the past two years. Duffy significantly expanded my perspective of the challenges facing the health care industry and provided me with a standard for excellence for which to strive.

Dr. Lois Friss, chairperson of my doctoral committee, who has provided me with a thought-provoking, sometimes skeptical perspective that has challenged my level of problem analysis.

Judy Baca, "my right arm," and Beverly Hartman, "my left arm," who have consistently provided me with the feedback and support I needed to be able to devote the time to such an endeavor.

Finally, the most important thanks goes to my husband, Peter, and son, Derek, for their continuous support and understanding during the writing of this book. To my husband for tolerating me bringing along my writing while waiting in between holes on the golf course, I thank you for never complaining. (Well, almost never!) To my son for typing and editing hundreds of pages of the manuscript on his Apple IIE, I thank you for being such a patient assistant. (Even though on one occasion you erased 100 pages of a chapter by putting one of your computer games on my diskette by mistake.)

It is only through the ongoing and unconditional support and love from special people in one's life that an individual can take the risk, and invest the time and energy to complete such as task. My heartfelt thanks to all of my "special people."

Contents

5   MARKETING SKILLS FOR NURSE ADMINISTRATORS   155

6   STRATEGIC PLANNING METHODS FOR NURSES   201

7   QUANTITATIVE METHODS AND DECISION MAKING   235

8 NETWORKING SKILLS FOR NURSES 283

9 POWER AND POLITICS FOR NURSE LEADERS 301

GLOSSARY 333

INDEX 339

Principles of Economics for Nurse Managers

THE ABILITY to understand the economic implications of the changing reimbursement system and the ability to forecast possible alternative futures are important skills for health care managers. Integration of these skills by managers will be necessary to anticipate change and implement meaningful and effective short-term and strategic plans for the successful health care organization.

The future of an acute care institution lies in its ability to cope with the rapidly changing marketplace and its environment. The time it takes an institution to respond to its environment is crucial for its survival in the increasingly competitive marketplace.

This chapter will outline basic economic principles to provide a framework for understanding economic theory, and then it will focus on the past, present, and future economics of the health care industry. The focus on the health care industry will include an outline of the historical economic environment that health care has experienced and details of current economic changes in the industry. The focus and perspective will be from the context of the nursing manager and/or administrator. Economic examples will include situations that nurse managers and/or administrators experience on a daily basis with hands-on examples of these concepts.

OBJECTIVES

Upon completing this chapter, the reader will be able to

1. Define and understand basic economic terminology.
2. Identify the major assumptions and relationships in economic theory.
3. Apply basic economic principles to the health care industry.
4. Define and understand the law of supply and demand.
5. Outline the economic changes in the health care industry during the past 30 years.
6. Identify ten driving trends currently affecting the health care industry.
7. Understand the impact of TEFRA and DRGs on the health care industry and nursing profession.
8. Identify four possible future scenarios for the health care industry.

BASIC ECONOMIC THEORY

Economic reality is an inescapable factor in the environment. The American College dictionary defines economics as "the science that treats production, distribution, and consumption of goods and services or the material welfare of mankind."[1] Economy is defined as "thrifty management; frugality in the expenditure or consumption of money, or materials, etc."[1] Both of these definitions include the components of goods and/or services and consumption of the same.

Weidenaar and Weiler defined economics as the "science of

managing scarcity."[2] They proposed that scarcity exists whenever resources are inadequate to meet the wants of a person or
society. The concept of scarcity limits the consumption and production of goods and drives the basic assumptions in economic
theory.

Goods are defined as tangible items that are produced to
meet consumers' wants or desires. *Services* are defined as
intangible items that are produced to meet consumers' needs or
wants. An example of a good is medication, whereas an example of a service is nursing care.

Goods and services are obtained through the exchange of
economic resources. Money is an example of such an economic
resource that can purchase or be exchanged for goods and services. Consumers obtain goods and services through their
income. *Income* is defined by the economist as all increases in
wealth plus consumption. Individuals receive income or wages
from the sale of their labor or services. This income is then used
to buy goods and services, or to save for the future.

The purchase of goods and/or services is termed *consumption*. This consumption of goods or services produces utility for
the individual. *Utility* is the term used to define the value of a
good or service to an individual or society. Value is a very
important concept in economics. *Value* is the worth of a good or
service as perceived by an individual or society. Value is not a
given. Things have value because people think they have
value. Value is a different concept for each individual, and
because individual perceptions of value differ, demand for particular goods and/or services varies.

Non-money income is the value of goods and services that
are not bought and sold in the marketplace and therefore do not
have a price tag. Examples of non-money income include the
value of a nurse's leisure time or time off, the value of clean air,
and the recreational value of a park or lake.

Robert Bingham stresses the concept of limited resources or
"scarcity," in his textbook, *Economic Concepts*.[3] He states that
the world is made up of people whose wants are greater than
their resources. This creates the concept of scarcity. Rich or
poor, people's wants always exceed their resources. This concept is the foundation for the discipline called economics.

The more resources an individual or an economy has access

to, the more wants or needs can be attained by the individual or the society. When an individual or society has limited access to resources, efficient use or management of resources becomes an important strategy to maximize the amount of goods or services one can attain. Maximum amounts of goods and services are obtained by either acquiring more resources or efficient management or utilization of limited resources. It is crucial to understand that the price one person pays for a good or service is the income of another person. It is possible to see that the concept of scarcity determines the ultimate consumption, production of services, and income of a society.

In a hospital setting, the hospital's access to resources determines its ability to produce health care services, the ability of the community to consume services, and its employees' income levels. In the current health care economic environment, this concept translates into the fact that a hospital's ability to grow or expand depends on its access to capital or money. Access to capital is the main reason many smaller, acute care institutions have recently joined larger multi-hospital chains.

ECONOMIC MODELS

Frequently, it is easier to understand a theory or concept when it is described in terms of a model. A model is a simplification or abstraction of reality. It includes the most important concepts of an idea or theory, and visually displays the inter-relationships of its parts. It is an abstract representation of the real thing. Blueprints of a hospital construction program are an example of a model.

The most popular model of economic theory is the neo-Keynesian model.[4] This model is based on the following assumptions:

Neo-Keynesian Assumptions

1. Individuals act to minimize pain and maximize pleasure.
2. All resources are limited, whereas wants are unlimited.
3. Play is pleasurable and work is painful.

The Neo-Keynesian economic model makes the following points based on those assumptions:

Postulates of Neo-Keynesian Economics

1. People would rather play than go to work.
2. People would rather possess goods (*e.g.*, cars or stereos) than live in a state of poverty.
3. There is a direct relationship between working and having material goods.
4. There is a relationship between being idle and living in poverty.
5. Individuals make trade-off decisions between the pleasure of play and the pain of poverty and the pleasure of possessing goods and the pain of work.
6. Not all individuals make the same decisions.

Supply Side of Economics

The classic supply side model of economics acknowledges that supply and demand determine the efficiency of an economy. The supply side of economic theory will be discussed first because supply has been the major focus in health care economics in the past.

The term *supply* is commonly used to define the quantity of a good or service present in the marketplace for consumers to purchase. This is the definition that most people, including consumers, associate with the term "supply." Economic theory postulates that when the supply of a commodity is high, the price decreases. This is called an inverted relationship.

A definition of supply that is more frequently used by economists is the "quantity of a good or service that would be offered or supplied at a particular price." Supply could be defined as a table or schedule of quantities of a particular commodity that the marketplace would offer at various prices. This definition of supply is from the perspective of the seller, whereas the first definition of supply was from the perspective of the purchaser. From the seller's perspective there is a direct relationship between the price at which a commodity is offered, and the quantity the seller is willing to supply in the marketplace.

A *marketplace* or *market* is the medium in which buyers and sellers interact to exchange goods and services for money. When an economy is a competitive economy, the marketplace sets the prices. In a noncompetitive economy such as the Soviet

Union, prices are set by the government rather than the marketplace. A market is not a geographical location like a grocery store. A market is created whenever buyers and sellers of a common product or service interact to exchange resources.

Price is defined as the ratio of exchange between two commodities. The price of a good or service is determined by the perceived value of the commodity.

It is important to keep in mind that the different definitions of supply result from the different perspectives involved. The first definition of supply is from the consumer's perspective and states that when there is a large supply of a commodity available, the price decreases. The second definition of supply is from the seller's perspective and states that when the seller can obtain a higher price for a commodity, he is willing to make available to the public a greater supply of the commodity. It is important to distinguish between the supply of a commodity and the quantity supplied because they have very different implications in economic theory.

SUPPLY THEORY IN HEALTH CARE

The traditional relationships between supply and price from the seller's perspective has had significant implications in the health care industry. The price of health care services has risen dramatically over the past 20 years, increasing the amount and kinds of services that health care providers are willing to offer. It is easy to see that when prices for health care services increase, health care providers are willing to offer more services. When it is possible to make a good profit on the sale of a good or service, the seller is willing to make more goods or services available so that he can make a bigger profit. This is an example of an economic explanation for the rapid rise in the availability or supply of health care services from the 1960s to the 1980s. Figure 1-1 shows this relationship of price and supply as applied to health care services. It is this relationship that has motivated hospitals to expand their capacities during the past 20 years.

The consumer's perspective of the relationship between supply and price has been almost nonexistent in the health care industry during the same period of time. In fact, the consumer had no thought for the price of health care services in the 1960s

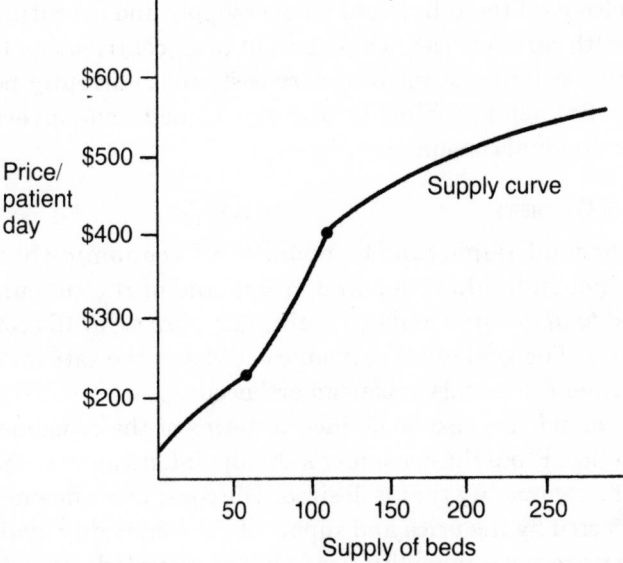

Figure 1-1. *Supply of health care services.*

and 1970s. This was true because the individual did not actually pay the bills and therefore had no concern for the price of health care services.

It is important to return to one of our original economic assumptions to understand this concept. The assumption is that individuals seek to maximize the utility of their resources. Because individual consumers did not have to produce the resources to pay for health care services, for the most part, they maximized their use of health care goods and services, without thinking about price or utility. They had, in essence, unlimited resources for their health care wants and needs.

We have said that, in reality, all resources are limited. The past economic environment in the health care industry, however, actually promoted gross overutilization of services because of the consumer's perception of unlimited resources. Efficiency was also not an issue in health care delivery, because health care institutions were reimbursed retrospectively based on their costs. With few exceptions, health care institutions were reimbursed their costs to deliver as many services as the consumer wished to receive.

The perception of having infinite resources because someone else paid the bill, led to an oversupply and overutilization of health care services. These are, in turn, contributing factors to the escalation of medical care costs that currently poses a major financial problem for the government, employers, and the individual consumer.

Demand Side of Economics

The second important component of economic theory is demand. Individual demand or demand of the consumer is called *final demand* and is the ultimate purpose of all economic activity. The goal of all economic activity is the satisfaction of consumers' demands or consumers' needs.

Demand can also be defined in terms of the consumer and the seller. From the consumer's standpoint, demand is the supply of a commodity that is desired. The consumer's demand will be affected by the price and supply of the commodity available. If the price of a commodity rises, the consumer's demand for the commodity usually falls. There is an inverted relationship between price and demand from the consumer's perspective.

Weidenaar and Weiler define *demand* as "a schedule of alternative quantities of a good or service that a person or group of people is willing to purchase at each alternative price during a specific period of time."[2] Factors that affect the demand for a good or service include the following:

1. The price of the service or goods
2. The price of closely related goods or services
3. Income
4. Wealth
5. Individual taste or preference
6. Perceptions of value

From a market standpoint, demand is the quantity of a commodity that will be demanded in the marketplace at various prices. As the price for a commodity increases, the demand for the same commodity decreases. In the case of demand, the same relationship between price and demand is true for both the marketplace and the consumer. This relationship is called the law of demand. The *law of demand* is the inverse relationship of price to quantity demand that exists for virtually all goods and services. This law states that as price decreases, quantity demanded increases. Conversely, as price of a commodity increases, quantity demanded decreases.

Elasticity is the measure of relative responsiveness of changes in quantity demanded to change in price. Demand is considered elastic if the quantity demanded changes more than the price changes. For example, a demand schedule for outpatient cataract surgeries could look like this:

Demand Schedule for Cataract Surgeries

Price/Surgery	Quantity Demanded (Cases)
$750	100
$1000	50
$1500	15

In this example, demand would be considered elastic because the demand for outpatient cataract operations decreased at a greater rate than the price increased. *Inelastic demand* results when the decrease in quantity demanded is smaller than the percentage of the increase in price. A demand schedule for emergency department visits shows that the change in quantity demanded is less than the increase in price. Emergency services are essentially inelastic because people who need the service are not significantly concerned about price.

Demand Schedule for Emergency Services

Price/Visit	Quantity Demanded (Visits)
$50	200
$150	200
$200	190
$300	180

The importance of the concept of elasticity lies in its ability to predict the effect that price increases or decreases will have on the quantities demanded in the marketplace. For example, outpatient cataract surgery has an elastic demand, or as price is increased by a specific amount the demand for the procedure will decrease at a greater rate. Cataract surgery can be considered very price sensitive. A hospital administrator would not want to raise the price significantly because that would result in a disproportionate decrease in the demand for the procedure in the marketplace.

Figure 1-2 shows graphically the relationship between price and demand for inpatient beds. Price is displayed along the vertical axis. It is possible to see the inverted relationship between price and demand on this graph. The line formed by the various quantities demanded at specific prices is called the *demand curve.*

Demand theory acknowledges that all resources are limited. Because of this price, becomes an issue in determining what is consumed or bought. Individuals make decisions about and trade-offs in their consumption of goods and services based on their perceptions of utility and price. Economic theory states that individuals purchase goods and services in a combination that maximizes their utility.

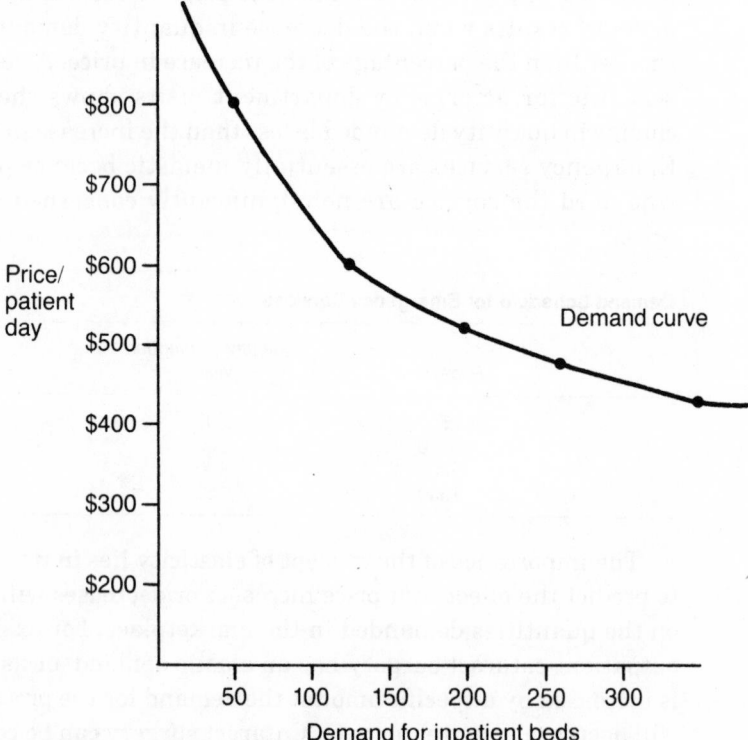

Figure 1-2. *Demand for inpatient services.*

DEMAND THEORY IN HEALTH CARE

Individuals purchase health care services that they perceive as providing utility or value to them at a price they can afford. Demand theory can be applied only to the health care industry in the 1950s, when the individual actually "purchased" his own health care services.

After the 1950s, third-party payors, industry, and the government became the purchasers of most health care services. The individual consumer was cut off from involvement in consumption choices. Health care services became separated from the demand component of economic theory because price was not an issue in the marketplace.

It is safe to say that during the past 20 years, the health care marketplace focused on the supply component of economic theory. When acknowledging the role demand plays in the results of economic competition, it must be remembered that there has been little competition in the health care field until recent years. Demand was not an issue because health care incentives were based on providing a greater supply of services. As long as the individual did not have to pay for the service, he had no incentive to "shop around" or make choices based on price or utility. As long as he did not have to pay for the service, he could "afford" to utilize a lot of services. Utilization of health care services skyrocketed to unbelievable proportions.

In the 1960s, third-party payors, industry, and the government replaced the individual as the real purchaser of health care services. As employers assumed the responsibility for their employees' health care coverage and benefits, the individual no longer consumed health care services based on his own perceptions of utility and price. Because full health care coverage was an employee benefit, there was no need to make trade-off decisions to maximize utility or minimize price.

The perception of unlimited health care services at no cost to the individual resulted in a focus on the supply of health care services available. Whoever could provide the greatest supply of services profited the most in the marketplace. The supply of health care services included volume as well as variety of services. Supply ruled the health care marketplace.

As supply increased, utilization skyrocketed and costs of health care services became prohibitive for the government, employers, and third-party payors. In reality, resources were not infinite, and something had to give. This is how the health care industry arrived at where it is today and why the government was pressured into a position where they needed to do something drastic. The government's response was to pass the Tax Equity Fiscal Responsibility Act (TEFRA) of 1982.

ECONOMIES OF SCALE

In the production of hospital services, labor or certain resources are utilized as inputs to produce patient care services, or outputs. Different levels of inputs produce varying levels of outputs at different costs per unit of output.[5] The concept of *economies of scale* identifies the optimal output or patient days that coincides with the lowest average cost per unit of service (UOS). This optimal level of output or number of patient days can be utilized to plan the number of beds that a hospital should have.

SAMPLE CALCULATIONS

Optimal number of patient days ÷ 365 days × budgeted occupancy = optimal number of beds for a hospital
43,800 Patient Days ÷ 365 days × 80% occupancy = 150 beds

For a hospital, economies of scale calculations identify the number of patient days and beds that can be offered to the community at the lowest average cost per patient day. In the current cost-conscious health care environment, this is an important concept.

When a hospital is very small, operating costs are high because of the small number of outputs or patient days over which fixed costs must be spread. Similarly when a hospital is very large, high management and administrative costs result in high unit costs or cost per UOS. Economies of scale describe the effects of the long-run average cost curve on volume for a business (Fig. 1-3).

The concept of economies of scale is very prevalent in planning for capacity in other industries. There has been some controversy, however, concerning whether the effect of economies of scale is a strong influence in the hospital because of its complexity.[5]

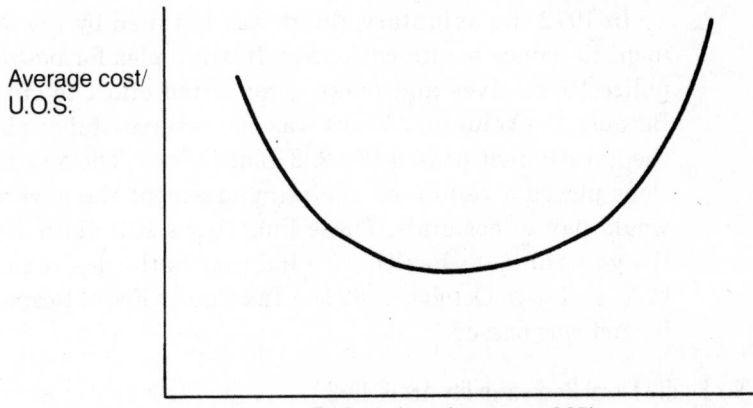

Figure 1-3. *Long run average cost curve.*

HISTORY OF THE MEDICARE PROGRAM

The Medicare Program began in 1965 under the Social Security System.[6] At that time the federal government was increasing the number of social programs it sponsored, and it seemed a given that the government should sponsor a health care plan for individuals that could not assume responsibility for their own health care needs. The Medicare Program was established to provide health care coverage and/or services for individuals who reached the age of 65 and/or became disabled. The program was originally structured so that the individual contributed to the program during his working years through Social Security payroll deductions. The individual would then receive health care benefits when he reached 65 and/or became disabled and could not afford his own health care coverage.

Medicare encountered a variety of problems, however. Double-digit inflation, overutilization of services, and a rapidly growing population increased the government's health care liability. It is important to understand that the government is the single largest consumer of all health care services in the United States. The federal government pays 60% to 70% of the total health care bills in the United States. One out of ten dollars the government spent in 1983 was for health care services. Because the government was paying the majority of all health care bills, it is easy to see why it had a vested interest in reducing the cost of health care.

In 1972 the Voluntary Effort was initiated by the government to reduce health care costs. It was a plea for hospitals to police themselves and make a concerted effort to cut costs. Because the Voluntary Effort was not as successful as planned, the government passed the 223 Limitations. The 223 Limitations placed a ceiling on the reimbursement the government would pay to hospitals. These limitations still did not reduce the government's health care liability to the desired magnitude, and so in October 1982 the Tax Equity Fiscal Responsibility Act was passed.

Tax Equity Fiscal Responsibility Act of 1982

Passage of the Tax Equity Fiscal Responsibility Act (TEFRA) of 1982 resulted in major changes for health care institutions. The reimbursement changes that went into effect on October 1982 included the following[7]:

- Elimination of the private room subsidy
- Elimination of Hill-Burton funds to hospitals
- Elimination of the anti-union subsidy for hospitals
- Reduction of hospital skilled nursing (SNF) per day rates by 50%
- Limits on the numbers of surgical assistants that Medicare would reimburse for a surgery
- Elimination of the 5% nursing differential
- Reductions in the amount of Medicaid payments the federal government would pay the states
- Limits on outpatient payments

In 1983 Congress passed the Social Security Amendments that included reimbursement by Diagnostic Related Group (DRG).[7] In the past, the health care industry had been reimbursed retrospectively. That is, reimbursement was determined after the actual services were delivered. For example, when a patient was admitted for an appendectomy, no one knew what the bill would be until the patient was discharged.

Prospective Reimbursement

Prospective reimbursement is reimbursement that is determined before the services are actually rendered. In a prospective reimbursement system, a hospital knows on admission the amount of money that will be reimbursed for a patient with an appendectomy, before the services are actually delivered. The Medicare DRG payment is a per discharge rate for the care rendered to a patient recovering from an appendectomy. It does not matter how long the patient stays in the hospital, how much laboratory work is ordered, or how many medications the patient is given. The hospital will be paid by the number of "recovered" appendectomy patients rather than by the number of treatments, medications, or hospital days.

It is important to remember that in prospective reimbursement, rates are determined before the services are actually rendered. There are two different forms of prospective reimbursement that currently affect the health care industry. They include the following:

1. Medicare's per discharge DRG reimbursement
2. Per diem reimbursement that is a flat per day rate

Per diem reimbursement is a flat per day rate that a hospital receives for a patient's care. Reimbursement is not necessarily related to his specific condition or the specific services that he receives. In the Western states, third-party payors are approaching hospitals to contract for competitive per day rates for any patient admitted to their institutions.

In 1983, California's MediCal Program adopted a flat per diem reimbursement system. MediCal requested that all California hospitals interested in caring for MediCal patients submit bids for a low per diem contract rate for any MediCal patient who was admitted to the institution for care.

This bidding process fostered much competition between California hospitals vying for MediCal contracts. Contracts were awarded to hospitals that bid per diem rates in the range of $400 to $600 per day. Contract hospitals are reimbursed at the per day rate times the number of days the patient is hospitalized.

SAMPLE CALCULATIONS

Per diem rate = $500/day
Hospitalization = ✕3 days
Total money reimbursed = $1500 to hospital

It is noteworthy that hospitals actually profit in a prospec-

•

tive per diem reimbursement situation by increasing the patient length of stay (LOS). For example, when a patient is admitted to an institution, cost to care for him in the first days usually exceeds the $500 per day reimbursement rate. This is because of the patient's need for admitting laboratory work, x-rays, EKGs, and aggressive nursing care and interventions. As the patient's condition improves, theoretically, the daily cost to care for the patient declines to the point of being less than the $500 per day reimbursement figure. If the hospital discharges the patient early, the hospital loses the revenue from the days when costs are below reimbursement. This profit margin acquired in the last few days of hospitalization is necessary to compensate for the losses incurred in the early days of the hospitalization. Figure 1-4 shows the profit and loss in per diem reimbursement and the relationship with LOS.

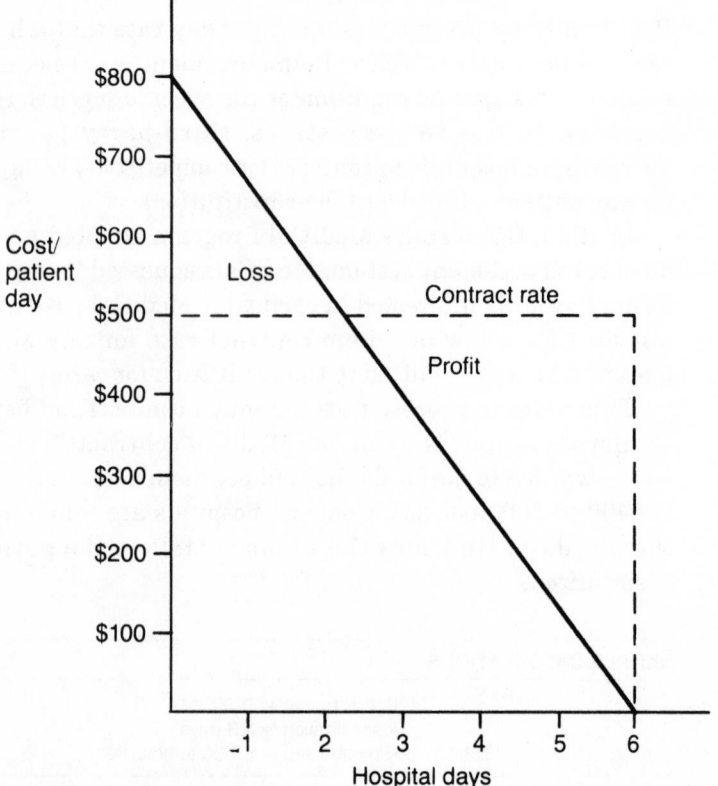

Figure 1-4.   *Per diem reimbursement analysis.*

Medicare DRGs

A DRG reimbursement system has been in effect in New Jersey since 1980, and in Maryland and New York since 1982,[8] having been implemented by these states on a voluntary basis in conjunction with the Yale Research Project, which first identified the concept of Diagnostic Related Groups. The Yale Research Project categorized 400,000 Medicare medical records into 23 Major Diagnostic Categories (MDCs) and then into 465 Diagnostic Related Groups (DRGs) using a decision tree methodology. The MDCs have medical significance, as shown in Table 1-1. It is important to note that DRGs are grouped by the fiscal resources utilized to "fix" a particular condition or disease. The impact of DRG reimbursement in these Eastern states has not been fully evaluated at this time because of the short time frame involved.

Table 1-1 shows the 23 MDCs that are in turn broken down into the 465 DRGs. Figure 1-5 shows the decision tree methodology of DRG assignment.

Table 1-1. Major Diagnostic Categories

Major Category	Group Description
1	Diseases and disorders of the nervous system
2	Diseases and disorders of the eye
3	Diseases and disorders of the ear, nose, and throat
4	Diseases and disorders of the respiratory tract
5	Diseases and disorders of the circulatory system
6	Diseases and disorders of the digestive system
7	Diseases and disorders of the hepatobiliary system
8	Diseases and disorders of the musculoskeletal system
9	Diseases and disorders of the skin, subcutaneous tissue and breast
10	Endocrine, nutritional, and metabolic diseases
11	Diseases and disorders of the kidney and urinary tract
12	Diseases and disorders of the male reproductive system
13	Diseases and disorders of the female reproductive system
14	Pregnancy, childbirth, and the puerperium
15	Newborns and other neonates
16	Diseases and disorders of the blood
17	Myeloproliferative disorders
18	Infectious and parasitic diseases
19	Mental diseases and disorders
20	Substance abuse
21	Injuries, poisonings, and toxic effects of drugs
22	Burns
23	Factors influencing health status and other contacts with health services

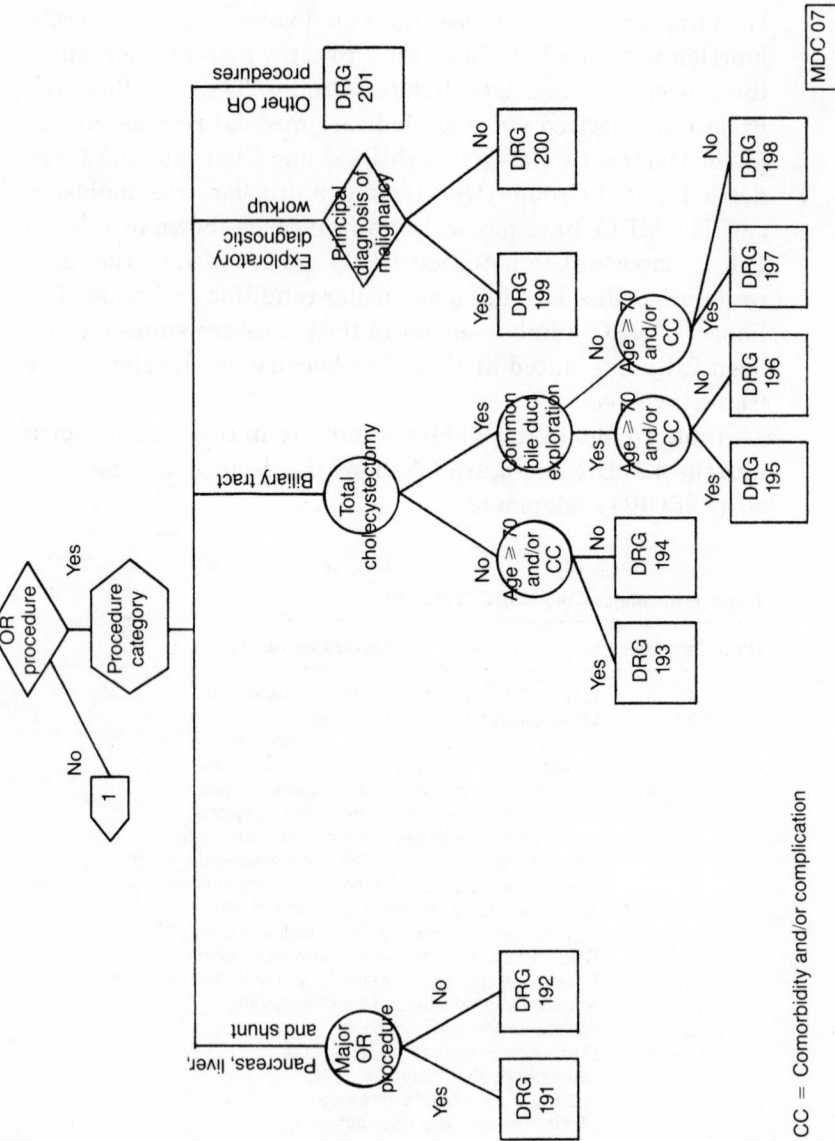

CC = Comorbidity and/or complication

Figure 1-5. Major diagnostic category 07: diseases and disorders of the hepatobiliary system and pancreas. Surgical partitioning.

EXAMPLE

If a patient is admitted to an institution for upper right quadrant pain and indigestion, he would be classified into MDC 07, diseases and disorders of the hepatobiliary system and pancreas. The first question on the decision tree that must be answered is as follows:

Was there an operating room procedure?

If the answer is yes, follow down that branch to the next question.

Did the operating room procedure involve the
• *Pancreas, liver, and shunt?*
• *Biliary tract?*
• *Exploratory?*
• *Other?*

If the answer is *surgery of the biliary tract* the next question is as follows:

Was the surgery a total cholecystectomy?

If the answer is *yes,* proceed down the branch to the next question:

Was a common bile duct exploratory included?

If the answer is *yes,* proceed down to the next question:

Was the patient over age 70 and/or have any complications or comorbidity?

The medical records department would note that the patient was 52 years old and that there were no complications, and code the patient DRG 196. this coding is transcribed onto the patient's Medicare billing form, which is sent to Medicare for payment. The flat DRG payment the hospital receives from Medicare is payment in full for the care of that patient, without regard to hospital costs. The hospital cannot bill the patient for the difference. The DRG payment is the total revenue the hospital receives for the patient's care.

The payment that the hospital receives is for the cholecystectomy patient who has recovered. The hospital is no longer reimbursed for treatments, medications, or x-rays per se. The service for which the hospital is reimbursed is the discharge of recovered patients, not the performance of procedures.

Exceptions to the flat per discharge rate from Medicare are called outliers. *Outliers* are patients that have a greater length of stay or unusually high cost of care compared with the average patient in that DRG according to the Yale Research Project. The specific days representing the high and low end of patient length of stay (LOS) are called *trim points*. Patients who are hospitalized longer than the trim point for a specific DRG are called *day outliers*. Patients who experience excessive costs for care without extending beyond the trim point are called *cost outliers*.

Hospitals are reimbursed by Medicare for day outliers and cost outliers at a reasonable cost-plus basis. This is not an automatic procedure, however. When an institution has a day or cost outlier, it must complete the necessary paperwork and request Medicare to visit the institution to review the patient chart for reimbursement as on outlier. Medicare may elect to decline the request or reimburse the hospital by the alternative method.

Cost outliers are calculated by identifying the TEFRA Target Rate and multiplying it by the relative cost weight for a specific DRG. If actual patient care costs exceed the maximum reimbursable rate for a specific DRG without reaching the high trim point, the hospital may approach Medicare for reimbursement as a cost outlier. (The TEFRA Target Rate will be calculated shortly.) The government acknowledges that DRG reimbursement is a drastic change for the health care industry and will have significant implications for the financial status of acute care institutions. Therefore, the DRG reimbursement system is being phased in over a 4-year period. Every hospital began this phasing-in period at the beginning of its first fiscal year after October 1983. If a hospital's financial year begins in October, that hospital started using DRGs from the very beginning, or October 1983. If a hospital has a fiscal year that begins in January, it started DRG reimbursement in January 1984.

The implementation timetable for DRG reimbursement was as follows[8]:

- 1983—Hospitals were reimbursed by Medicare at reasonable cost subject to 223 Limitations and TEFRA limits.
- 1984—75% of Medicare reimbursement was according to the TEFRA Target Rate, and 25% was according to the flat DRG rate.
- 1985—50% of Medicare reimbursement was at the TEFRA Target Rate and 50% by flat DRG rate.
- 1986—25% of Medicare reimbursement is by the TEFRA Target Rate, and 75% by flat DRG rate.
- 1987—100% of Medicare payments are based on flat DRG rates (separate rural and urban rates for each DRG).

TEFRA Target Rate

The government realized that the reimbursement changes would have drastic economic implications for acute care institutions and wanted to allow acute care providers ample time to make the necessary changes to the expense side of their operations in order to cope with the decreases on the revenue side. Consequently, hospitals were to receive three different hospital-specific adjustments during a transitional period. The hospital-specific adjustments for the 4-year transitional period include the following[9]:

1. Wage adjustment
2. Educational adjustment
3. Case mix index adjustment

The government understands that not all hospitals experience the same expenses. Specifically, labor costs vary greatly from one area of the country to another and from large institutions to small institutions. The government is not interested in regulating salaries or cost of living across the nation. Therefore, the average labor cost in acute care institutions across the nation was identified and assigned a *wage index* of 1.0. Individual hospital wages were then compared with the average wage index, and each hospital was given a hospital-specific wage index.

If a hospital paid higher than average salaries, the hospital received a wage index greater than 1.0. If a hospital paid lower than average salaries, the hospital received a wage index less than 1.0 (*e.g.*, .8 or .9).

If the national average hourly wage for acute care employees was calculated at $10 and a hospital paid an average wage of $12 per hour to its employees, their wage index wage is calculated like this:

CALCULATIONS

Hospital salary rate ÷ national average = wage index
$12/hour ÷ $10/hour = 1.2 wage index

If a hospital paid an average of $9 per hour, it received a wage index of .9.

CALCULATIONS

Hospital salaries ÷ national average salary = wage index
$9/hour ÷ $10/hour = .9 wage index

The second adjustment that hospitals receive is an *educational adjustment*. The government wants to support hospitals that continue medical and nursing education programs. This adjustment applies to off-site university- or college-based nursing and medical programs. It does not include inservice educational programs. The government evaluated education programs in hospitals across the nation and developed a profile for an average hospital-based nursing and medical program, assigning it an educational index of 1.0. Individual hospitals were compared with the profile and assigned an educational index based on the hours of residency, intern, and nursing programs in the institution.

If a hospital had an index greater than the national average, it was assigned an educational index greater than 1.0. Likewise, if its index was less than the national average, it received an educational index less than 1.0.

The final adjustment that institutions receive in the transitional period is the *case mix index*. The case mix index quantifies the complexity, intensity, and resources required to care for a specific patient population. The case mix index was identified by looking at all Medicare patients treated in the United States and determining the "average" mix of patients for an acute care institution. The average case mix of patients across 731the nation was assigned a 1.0 case mix index. It is important to note that the case mix index is a measure of the complexity and/or intensity of the care needed for a patient population in a particular acute care institution.

Each hospital's Medicare patient population was then compared with the average case mix and assigned a specific case mix index. If a hospital treated more complicated Medicare patients than the average, it received a case mix index greater than 1.0. If a hospital treated less complicated Medicare patients, it received a case mix index less than 1.0.

The statistics used to identify an institution's case mix index were gathered from 1979 to 1982. If a hospital's patient population or services change drastically, there are provisions to effect changes in the case mix index. This is a rather rigorous and difficult process, however, and can be done only once.

Using these adjustments, it is possible to calculate the TEFRA Target Limit for hospital-specific reimbursement in the transitional period. The TEFRA Target Limit is calculated by starting with the old 223 Limitations and adding the three adjustments.

SAMPLE CALCULATIONS

223 Limitation for acute MI	= $8000
Labor portion of bill	= ×.8
Labor portion of acute MI	= $6400
Hospital's Wage Index	= ×1.2
Wage adjusted reimbursement	= $7680
Supply portion of bill	= +$1600
Total wage adjusted reimbursement	= $9280
Educational adjustment	= +$200
Education adjusted limit	= $9480
Hospital's case mix index	= ×1.5
TEFRA Target Rate	= $14,220

When this specific hospital cares for an acute myocardial infarction (MI) in its first year using DRGs, the amount the hospital is reimbursed for this patient's care is based on 25% of the flat DRG rate and 75% of the TEFRA Target Rate.

When the TEFRA Target Rate for acute MI (DRG 122) is $14,220 and the flat DRG rate is $5500, the hospital would be reimbursed for this patient in 1984-85 as follows:

CALCULATIONS

TEFRA Target Rate × 25% = TEFRA Target portion

$14,220 = TEFRA Target Rate
× .75 = 1984–85 percentage
$10,665 = TEFRA Target amount

Flat DRG rate × 75% = DRG portion
$5500 = DRG rate
× .25 = 1984–85 percentage
$1375 = DRG portion

TEFRA Target portion + DRG portion = 1984–85 reimbursement
$10,665 + $1375 = $12,040 reimbursement for acute MI in 1984–85

Reimbursement for this same Acute MI patient in 1985-86 would decrease based on the transitional period percentages outlined previously. Reimbursement for 1985-86 is calculated as follows:

CALCULATIONS

TEFRA Target Rate × 50% = TEFRA Target portion

$14,220 = TEFRA Target rate for acute MI
× .50 = 1984–85 percentage
$ 7,110 = TEFRA Target portion

DRG Rate × 50% = DRG portion
$5,500 = DRG rate
× .50 = 1984–85 percentage
$2,750 = DRG portion

TEFRA Target portion + DRG portion = 1984–85 reimbursement
$7,110 + $2,750 = $9,860 reimbursement for 1984–85

Reimbursement for any specific DRG decreases from one year to the next in the transitional period until the reimbursement is a flat per DRG rate. After the transitional period, there will be only two different DRG rates per DRG. These two rates will be for rural and urban acute care institutions and will not be institution specific. Institutions will have a 4-year period during which to reduce their expenses. After the 4-year transitional period, hospitals will no longer receive hospital-specific adjustments for wages, education, and case mix.

Prospective Contracting

DRG prospective reimbursement has a significant impact on the revenue of acute care institutions. This impact is not limited to the Medicare patient population. Third-party payors and the Medical program in many states have also implimented reimbursement by DRG.

The second type of prospective reimbursement affecting the industry is per diem reimbursement. Many third-party payors are adopting this form of reimbursement. Institutions need to assess a number of factors when considering contracting and specific contract rates. As mentioned previously, the major way an institution profits from a per diem reimbursement system is by increasing the length of stay. In an environment of decreasing inpatient census, contracting is an important strategy to maintain inpatient census figures. Contract rates usually result in a reduced profit margin, but a patient in a bed contributes more than does an empty bed to the overhead costs of operating the hospital. Hospitals need to evaluate carefully the advantages and disadvantages of per diem contracting. It is predicted that within a few years a majority of third party-payors will be negotiating per diem or per discharge contracts with all acute care institutions. There are several important considerations in determining an institution's ability to benefit and/ or survive with per diem and per discharge contracts. These considerations include the following:

- The institution's case mix profile
- The institution's current payor profiles
- The institution's fiscal health
- The percentage of patients that would be reimbursed by the per diem and/or per discharge rates
- The specific per diem and/or per discharge contract rates
- The hospital's average LOS per diagnosis
- The institution's ability to manage efficiently
- The institution's physician practice patterns and relationship with the institution

There are risks associated with both contracting and not contracting. The risks associated with contracting include inability to make a bottom-line profit with the contracting rates, increased LOS, and increasing patient complications resulting from expense reductions. The risk associated with not contracting is a steadily declining inpatient census.

Peer Review Organizations

In 1983, Congress repealed the Professional Standards Review Organization Program. Now hospitals will contract with for-profit or nonprofit Peer Review Organizations (PROs) to perform their utilization review.

These Peer Review Organizations are composed of licensed physicians and nurses practicing in the area, who are familiar with the community standards of care. They review services provided to Medicare beneficiaries for medical necessity and appropriateness of the admission.

To understand the full impact of the review process, the criteria the PROs utilize include the following[9]:

- Five percent of all routine Medicare records are reviewed.
- All outliers are reviewed.
- All transfers to any other acute care facility are reviewed.
- All readmissions are reviewed.
- All fatalities are reviewed.
- All admissions within 7 days of discharge from an acute care facility are reviewed.
- Loss of JCAH will be reviewed.
- All invasive procedures are reviewed for medical necessity.

- Review of records may occur at any time with less than 24 hours notice.

- All documentation to validate the DRG assignment is reviewed.

- Studies and treatments are reviewed for appropriateness to the principal diagnosis.

The initial review standard of 5% of all Medicare charts is a misleading figure. When hospitals total their incidence of fatalities, readmissions, transfers, and so on, the actual percentage of charts that is reviewed by the PROs equals 40% to 60% of the Medicare charts. This is a significant number of charts.

Principal Diagnosis

A final concept in the DRG reimbursement system is that all hospital cases will be assigned one DRG code based on *principal diagnosis*. There are three different types of diagnoses commonly used in the acute care setting. The first is called the *admitting diagnosis*. The definition of admitting diagnosis is "the most likely cause for the patient's admission to the institution."

The second diagnosis is the *primary diagnosis*. The primary diagnosis is "the condition that best describes the services the patient receives while in the hospital." This is frequently very different or even unrelated to the admitting diagnosis.

The third type of diagnosis is the *principal diagnosis*. The principal diagnosis is "the diagnosis that best describes, after study, the condition that caused the patient to come into the hospital in the first place." The phrase "after study" is the most important part of the third definition because it can be determined only at discharge.

Medicare DRG reimbursement is based only on the principal diagnosis. Medicare is not concerned with what the physician "thought" was wrong with the patient and recorded in the admitting diagnosis or what the patient was treated for after being admitted to the hospital. Medicare will reimburse only for the principal diagnosis or for the condition that caused the patient to be admitted to the institution.

SAMPLE CASE

A patient is admitted to an acute care institution with acute right sided chest pain. His admitting diagnosis is "rule out myocardial infarction." He is placed in the CCU and monitored for 48 hours and then found to have negative enzymes and no EKG changes. The patient is moved to the medical–surgical unit and worked up for a duodenal ulcer, cholecystitis, and so on. The patient's primary diagnosis is then identified as duodenal ulcer because of his 3 days of medical treatment. On the 6th day of hospitalization, the patient grows worse, and an emergency laparotomy is performed. The surgery reveals that the patient had a pancreatic tumor, which was surgically removed. The reimbursement the institution receives for this patient will be based on the principle diagnosis of pancreatic tumor. The institution will be reimbursed only for that procedure and condition and will receive nothing for the medical interventions to rule out MI or duodneal ulcer.

The economic environment of the health care industry and the reimbursement changes outlined here have a significant impact on the fiscal health of all acute care institutions. Only institutions that have knowledge of that impact and its implications, and an ability to respond quickly will survive. It is in this area that effective nursing managers and administrators will truly make a difference for their institution's survival.

ECONOMIC FORECASTING

Forecasting is a method of determining what may happen in the future based on current driving trends. After potential future events are identified, the process of strategic planning is utilized to bring about the desired future. The strategic planning process is outlined in detail in Chapter Six and will not be discussed further here. The management tool of forecasting is discussed for the purpose of identifying alternative economic scenarios that will influence the health care industry in the future.

The future is not a matter of chance but rather a matter of choice. This choice involves forecasting potential scenarios and then selecting the desired future based on the organization's mission statement and goals. This process includes the following steps:

1. Identify the organization's present position.
2. Identify the organization's weaknesses and strengths.
3. Identify the driving trends in the environment that could be threats or opportunities for the organization.
4. Construct possible alternative future scenarios based on the driving trends in the environment.
5. Identify the desired future for the organization.

Future Socioeconomic Scenarios

After scanning the environment for years, John Naisbitt outlined ten driving trends in his popular book *Megatrends*.[10] These trends include the following:

1. Information society
2. High tech/high touch
3. World economy
4. Long-term perspective
5. Decentralization
6. Self-help
7. Participatory democracy
8. Networking
9. Southern migration
10. Multiple options

Naisbitt's book has significantly contributed to increasing the awareness of forecasting as a useful management tool. Forecasting has only recently been utilized in the health care field. A new discipline called futures research acknowledges the necessity of identifying possible future scenarios to select the desired future. The next step is for the institution to develop and implement a strategic plan to reach that future. The discipline scans the environment for driving trends that could be indicators of the future. One method futurists use to identify possible futures is called *scenario writing,* in which they combine projections, assumptions, and forecasts of current trends to create potential future scenarios or stories. The Lutheran Hospital Society's Center for Health Management Research has on its staff one of the first health care futurists, who has been actively involved in writing scenarios. This futurist, Russell Coile, headed the Lutheran Hospital Society's Health Network of America Futures Program and wrote about the following four socioeconomic scenarios for the health care industry[11]:

Scenario One: Continued growth or boom

Scenario Two: Competition or conglomerates

Scenario Three: Decline and stagnation

Scenario Four: Voluntary simplicity or transformation

Health care futurists identified these scenarios using the ten driving forces in the health care industry in the 1980s, which include the following[11]:

1. Aging
2. Competition
3. Conglomerates
4. New consumer
5. Corporate practice
6. Diversification
7. Information/telecommunications
8. Shifting dollars
9. Technopush
10. Changing values

Table 1-2 shows these ten driving forces, the scenarios they drive, and their economic implications for the future of the health care industry.

The Program Planning Committee of the California Hospital Association completed an in-depth assessment of the environment for the specific purpose of assisting hospitals to be able to plan for the changing health care environment. Specific economic concepts derived from that report will assist the reader in understanding the implications and magnitude of the changes ahead in the health care industry (Table 1-3).

SUMMARY

The health care industry is rapidly approximating the private for-profit sector. Nurse managers and administrators need to become knowledgeable and to acquire expertise in the economic realities affecting patient care delivery systems. The significant changes in the health care industry and economic concepts outlined in this chapter include the following:

1. The health care industry was driven by the economic factor of supply in the 1960s and 1970s as a result of retrospective cost-based reimbursement. Retrospective cost-based reimbursement created incentives for hospitals to develop a great variety and supply of health care services that were paid for by employers and the federal government.
2. Health care costs escalated uncontrollably during the 1960s and 1970s because of inflation, overutilization of

(Text continues on p. 32.)

Table 1-2. Driving Forces in the Health Care Industry

Driving Force	Affected Scenario	Health Care Implications
1. Aging	1, 2, 3, & 4	There will be increasing numbers of elderly consumers demanding specialized services. The need for chronic degenerative disease and organ transplantation services will increase, because of longer life expectancy. The market for an entire line of geriatric services will expand (*e.g.*, life care concept). Aggressive treatment modalities will be utilized in individuals much older than is now the case. Middle-aged persons will be 60 to 80 years old.
2. Competition	1, 2, & 3	Health care advertising will increase. Hospitals will compete with physicians and other health professionals for market. Increased numbers of hospitals and services will merge into conglomerates for strength. Health care consumers will shop around for services and price. Institutions will compete through pricing.
3. Conglomerates	1 & 2	The trend will be toward multi-hospital systems to accomplish economies of scale and increase power base. There will be a trend toward vertical integration, rather than full-service institutions. Health care institutions will "unbundle" services and diversify into other areas (*e.g.*, providing hotel services and rooms for visitors and community). There will be a trend toward joint venturing with competitors, physicians, nurses, and the public sector.
4. New consumer	1, 2, & 4	Consumers will be healthier, more price conscious, better educated, and informed about treatments and alternatives to maintaining their health. Consumers will take more responsibility for their own health and well-being. They will seek professional services less frequently than in the past. More books and audio and video recordings will be marketed, allowing the consumer to treat himself. The consumer will question the health care provider more frequently about the service and will demand more efficiency and greater quality.
5. Corporate practice	1, 2, 3, & 4	Diagnosing will be done by more cost effective and accurate computers. Cost and oversupply of physicians will motivate them to unite for economic security and power. They will create corporations to provide health care services in competition with hospitals.

Table 1-2. *(Continued)*

Driving Force	Affected Scenario	Health Care Implications
		Physicians will attempt to regulate health care policy by increasing lobbing activities.
		Physicians will become more generalist-minded to maintain clients. They will return to making house calls and be more sensitive and in-tune with consumer needs as a result of economic pressures.
6. Diversification	1, 2, & 4	There will be a great increase in the development of health care products (*e.g.*, vitamins, food, education, etc.).
		There will be a trend toward "unbundling" of hospital services and creating for-profit corporations (*e.g.*, incorporating the printing department and selling service to the community).
		There will be an increasingly broad re-definition of the "health care" business. The business will include services that improve the quality of life, rather than just treating illness.
		Joint ventures with physicians and nurses, and for-profit and public sector will increase.
		In the "information age," health information will be a business. Health information will include software to diagnose illness and prescribe treatment.
7. Information/tele-communications	1, 2, & 4	Diagnosis and prescription will be done by computers. Software for home personal computers will be available for sale.
		There will be the potential for a health care corporation to serve the world rather than a single community.
		Health care will become more a business of health information rather than actual hands-on care.
		All health care services will be capable of being delivered to the individual consumer's home.
8. Shifting dollars	1, 2, 3, & 4	The uncertain economic environment will create a three-tier health system:
		Public beneficiaries
		Middle class
		Wealthy
		The consumer will be willing to take more risk and responsibility for his own health. He will pay less for health care insurance by assuming a larger deductible.
		More health care institutions will become for-profit.
		There will be an increased demand for outpatient, home health services, etc.
		There will be decreased health care services available for the poor.

(continued)

Table 1-2.   *(Continued)*

Driving Force	Affected Scenario	Health Care Implications
9. Technopush	1 & 2	Life expectancy, productivity, and population will increase. The cost of health care will increase because of increased cost of research and development and increased number of people to care for. The number and complexity of ethical issues will increase as a result of high technology. The high tech aspect will be balanced by a corresponding development of high touch technology. Health care policy will be unable to keep up with the demands placed on it. Legal implications will become very complex in this high tech environment.
10. Values	1, 2, & 4	The complexity of bioethical issues will increase. There will be an increased number of arbitrations necessary among doctors, families, lawyers, and patients. Resource allocations may be determined on the cost-effectiveness of various health programs based on years of additional life provided. Many conflicts based on values will arise because of the diversity of ethnic groups in the United States.

services, increased rate of population growth, and the inefficiency of too many hospitals.

3. The federal government is the single largest consumer of health care services, paying 60% to 70% of all health care bills.

4. The law of supply and demand is the major concept in economic theory that identifies schedules for specific supply and demand at varying pricing levels. Supply varies directly with price.

5. Prospective reimbursement refers to payment schedules that are established before services are delivered. Examples of prospective reimbursement in health care include DRG or per discharge reimbursement and per diem contracting. Per discharge reimbursement is a flat fee for an entire hospital admission, whereas per diem contract rates are flat per day rates for inpatient care irrespective of diagnosis.

6. Individuals seek to maximize the value and utility of their

Table 1-3. Excerpts from Strategic Planning Assumptions for Hospitals 1984–1986

- More risk will be transferred to hospitals and physicians through the prospective rate system.

- Failing volume, high interest rates, and increased bad debts will be troublesome for hospitals until pent-up demand becomes evident.

- Economic priorities will move away from health care and inpatient hospital services.

- There will be a need for all hospitals to establish realistic profit objectives and profit margins.

- The Reagan administration proposals are fragmented, some favoring "competition" and others "regulation." These are piecemeal attacks. There is no unified national health policy, and there will not be one for years to come.

- The proportion of the U.S. population that is over the age of 65 will continue to increase; especially rapid increases are expected in the number of persons over the age of 75.

- Hospital capacity will be shown to be in excess of available revenue, resulting in either retirement or "mothballing" of presently licensed beds, closures, or conversations.

- Home care will become a growing issue as inpatient revenues become more controlled by negotiated contracts.

- Increases in the aged population will mean an increase in the need for intermediate or long-term care facilities, raising issues about the need for hospitals.

- With changing public interests and shifts in funding, there will be a greater emphasis on fitness, diet, and illness prevention.

- The number of specialized limited-purpose institutions providing services for a particular patient population will increase.

- There will be an increase in the number of hospital sponsored and managed ambulatory surgery, home care, and visiting nurse programs.

- Health Maintenance Organizations (HMOs) and Preferred Provider Organizations (PPOs) will increase in prevalence and enrollment.

- Various contractural mechanisms will emerge offering bidding and competition for favorable groups of patients.

- High-medical risk, high financial risk patients will find increasing difficulty in obtaining services and coverage.

- Some public hospitals will not survive and will be sold or leased to priviate operations or will be closed.

- The financial aspect of hospital operations will continue to be the focal point of two countervailing forces:
  — Increasing pressures to contain costs
  — Financial ability of hospitals to adapt to the new competitive environment represented by negotiated contracts

- Cutbacks in federal support for major health programs will put great pressure on the states to shift the burden onto providers and individuals.

- Demand for review will continue to come from non-physicians, payors, or insurers. Physicians and hospitals will be forced to respond.

- There will continue to be a shift from federal to state level regulation of health care.

- There will be an increasing concern over the value of technology both in terms of economic costs and social value.

(Mitchell F: Strategic Planning Assumptions for Hospitals, 1984–1986. Program Planning Committee of the California Hospital Association, December 1983) resources. They make economic choices and purchases based on their perceptions of value and utility.

7. In a competitive marketplace, prices are determined by the market. As competition in health care increases, the marketplace rather than regulation will determine prices.

8. The DRG system is being phased in over a 4-year period. Hospital specific adjustments for case mix, wages, and education will be phased out by fiscal year 1987.

9. In 1983 the Professional Standard Review Organizations were repealed by Congress and replaced by Professional Review Organizations for utilization review.

10. DRG reimbursement is based totally on the principal diagnosis or the condition that best describes, after study, the reason that the patient needed inpatient care. The Medicare DRG payment is payment in full to the hospital. The hospital cannot bill the patient or family for any costs exceeding the DRG payment.

11. Forecasting is a method of identifying potential future scenarios based on the current driving trends in the environment. The driving trends currently affecting the health care industry include aging, competition, conglomerates, new consumers, corporate practice, diversification, changing values, information/telecommunications, shifting dollars, and technopush.

REFERENCES

1. American College Dictionary, 22nd ed. New York, Random House, 1968
2. Weidenaar DJ, Weiler ET: Economics: An Introduction to the World Around You. Reading, MA, Addison-Wesley, 1976
3. Bingham RC: Economic Concepts: A Programmed Approach. New York, McGraw-Hill, 1984
4. Graham P: Managerial Economics. Reading, MA, Addison-Wesley, 1980
5. Rapoport J, Robertson R, Stuart B: Understanding Health Economics. Rockville, MD, Aspen Publishers, 1982
6. Torrens PR: The American Health Care System: Issues and Problems. St Louis, CV Mosby, 1978
7. Grimaldi PL: Public Law 97-248: The implication of prospective payment schedules. Nurs Manage 14(2) Feb 1983
8. Grimaldi P, Micheletti J: DRG'S: A Practitioner's Guide. Chicago, Pluribus Press, 1983
9. Managing Medicare Prospective Pricing. Chicago, American Hospital Association Publication, 1983
10. Naisbitt J: Megatrends. Warren Books, 1984
11. Mitchell F, Cloner A, Coile R: Multi-scenario forecasting and

health management in the 1980's. Presented at the Third International Symposium on Forecasting in Philadelphia, June 6, 1983

ADDITIONAL READINGS

1. Changing Health Care Policy U.S.A, 1982. Concord, MA, International Health Sciences, 1982
2. Medicare Payment: Cost per Case Management Special Reports. Chicago, August 1983

Financial Management

HISTORICALLY, the need for competent financial management skills in the health care industry has taken a back seat to other goals, including quality patient care, increased levels of technology, and improved access to medical care for all people. In the 1980s, however, the health care institution's ability to maintain a strong financial position will determine the institution's ability to survive to provide *any* health care services at all.

In the case of the for-profit or private sector, financial management has always been a valued management skill. Successful financial managers are concerned with maximizing the institution's financial health and market position. In the private sector, that goal benefits the shareholders. In the not-for-profit or third sector, that goal allows the health care institution to survive, expand, and improve its services. The goal of maximizing the institution's financial position and strength somehow seemed unethical in the not-for-profit sector. The goal of maintaining fiscal health can be considered an appropriate goal, since all the profits are utilized to provide additional technology, programs, and services for the community. In the not-for-profit sector, all profits or wealth is to be utilized by the institution to expand or improve services, rather than being distributed among shareholders as in the private sector. The major difference between the for-profit and not-for-profit sectors can be explained by the use of profits.

The for-profit sector distributes profits to its shareholders, whereas the not-for-profit sector retains all profits within the company to improve and/or expand services.

Historically, not-for-profit health care institutions have set their financial or bottom-line goals for minimal profits. Many health care institutions in the not-for-profit sector actually budget for operating margins as low as 1% to 4%, whereas for-profit institutions budget operating margins at about 10% to 15%. *Operating margin* is the profit the institution realizes from operations, divided by the net patient revenues. *Net patient revenues* are the revenues the institution actually receives from patient care services after allowances and deductions are taken into account.

EXAMPLE

Revenues − expenses = profits ÷ net patient revenues = operating margin
$32,000 − $28,000 = $4,000 ÷ $28,200 = 14%

This example shows a healthy operating margin of 14%. When institutions budget for low operating margins, that margin can erode even lower if any unplanned expenses occur or patient revenues fall short of their budgeted projections. The not-for-profit sector has viewed the 10% to 15% operating margins in the for-profit sector as being "mercenary" and too "business-oriented" for a health care institution. The for-profit institutions merely consider themselves productive and efficient. They have operated more along the lines of other private industries, establishing specific goals for their financial performance.

This chapter will introduce basic financial management terminology, concepts, and strategies, all of which are becoming increasingly important to responsible health care managers in the performance of their job. Health care managers are being held more and more responsible and accountable for the fiscal management of their unit, department, and/or institution. Health care administrators are realizing the importance of maintaining the financial health and position of the organization. The single most important objective for the institution in this current environment is to have more financial resources coming into the facility than are going out. If this simple objective is not met, all other objectives are meaningless.

The profession of nursing has not been very concerned about financial management skills in the past. Therefore, as we find ourselves in an environment in which this is an important concern, it is vital that nurse managers and administrators equip themselves with the financial skills and expertise to assume this challenge. Because of the sheer size of the nursing department and its budget in all hospitals, it is more important for nursing managers to possess skills in financial management, than any other managers in the institution. Nursing staff, patients, and the institution itself will benefit from the application of these skills and expertise by nurse executives and managers.

OBJECTIVES

Upon completing this chapter, the reader will be able to

1. Define and utilize basic financial terminology.
2. Understand and analyze an income statement and balance sheet.
3. Identify and understand basic financial ratios.
4. Identify and understand various methods of capital financing.

5. Identify at least two methods of improving cash flow in a health care institution.
6. Understand the relationship between credit policy and accounts receivable management.
7. Define two different methods of managing inventories.

FINANCIAL ORGANIZATION OF THE HOSPITAL

The organizational structure of an institution can contribute to or detract from its efficiency and operations. There is no one ideal organizational structure recommended for hospitals. Various models are effective, depending on the size and characteristics of the organization, as well as the style of leadership and management of the institution.

In the 1980s, hospitals are reorganizing for financial and operational reasons. Many institutions have undergone reorganization more than once. This trend of reorganization is not necessarily detrimental, although reorganization can prove to be very traumatic and unsettling for organizational members when it occurs frequently in the same institution. Frequent changing of reporting relationships and job descriptions create an unsettling, unpredictable environment in which individuals begin to feel insecure.

According to Peters and Waterman, on the other hand, the sign of a progressive organization is its ability to change and be flexible in a changing environment with changing consumer demands[1]. It is important for an organization to be able to reorganize and/or change in response to its environment and consumers. However, because reorganization causes disruption within the organization, reorganization measures should be well thought out and implemented to accomplish a particular financial or operational goal. Once implemented, the administration needs to manage the disruption to minimize the negative impacts on the organization in obtaining its future financial and production goals.

The health care institution is financially and operationally accountable to the governing body or the board of directors. Figure 2-1 shows a typical organizational structure for a not-for-profit health care institution and the financial responsibilities and reporting relationships.

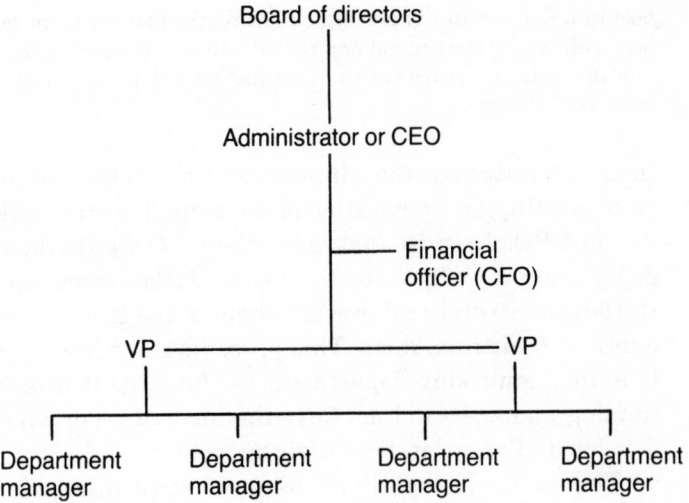

Figure 2-1. *Health care organizational structure.*

The board is responsible and accountable for all hospital activities and operations, as well as its financial performance. The board delegates actual management of operations to line administrative staff. The actual financial management of the institution is delegated to the administrator or chief executive officer (CEO) by the board. There is usually a board committee that focuses on the financial management of the hospital in conjunction with the administrator. This is usually called the finance committee of the board, and acts as the control mechanism for the board on hospital financial matters.

The finance committee is usually chaired by the hospital treasurer, who is not employed by the hospital. He or she is a voluntary member of the board and thus provides a system of checks and balances in conjunction with the hospital chief financial officer (CFO) or vice president (VP) of finance. The CFO or VP of finance is a hospital employee who is responsible for the hospital's day-to-day financial operations.

The Joint Commission on Accreditation for Hospitals has established the basic standards for the financial management of hospitals[2]:

The governing body, through its chief executive officer, shall provide for the control and use of the physical and financial resources of the hospital. Responsibility for implementing the policies of the governing body relative to the control and the effective utilization of the physical and financial resources of the hospital should be given to the chief executive officer.

In most institutions the administrator has delegated the major responsibility for preparation of the annual operational budget to the CFO. In most instances the CFO would develop all departmental budgets for the institution in conjunction with the administrator and present them to the department managers in their final form. This procedure has been especially true in the nursing department in the past. It was felt that nursing managers did not have the inclination or expertise to develop and/or understand their budgets.

This policy is rapidly changing in most institutions, and this change usually results in a more accurate and realistic budget. As the industry is becoming more concerned with efficiency and productivity, it is very appropriate and efficient for nursing as well as other department managers to develop their own budgets from the ground up. When managers develop their own budgets using parameters set by the CFO, they are more committed to them and can better understand the impact of various decisions on their own budgets.

This recent change in philosophy provides the major motivation for writing this chapter. It is believed that when nursing managers develop skills and expertise in budget preparation and financial management, the institution will be capable of improved decision making and productivity. The professional nurse will be capable of a higher level of performance and satisfaction in the management of patient care services. Career advancement is also improved for the nurse manager who develops these skills.

Other functions and responsibilities of the CFO include the following:

1. Planning the institution's overall budget operations
2. Recording and summarizing all financial transactions of the institution
3. Measuring and evaluating actual fiscal performance against budgeted performance
4. Facilitating communications regarding the institution's

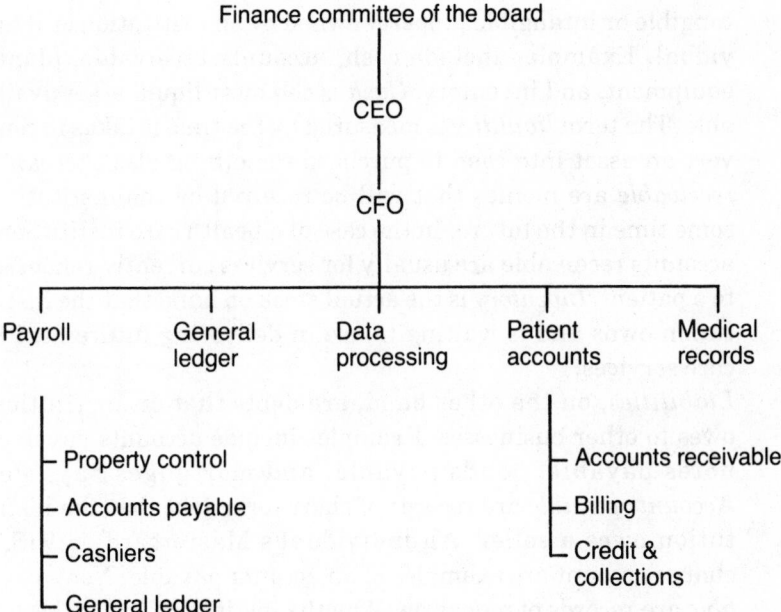

Figure 2-2. *Organization of financial services.*

financial status and performance to all levels of management and administration

Figure 2-2 shows a typical organizational structure of the financial service functions that report to the CFO. Note that the medical records department or function is the responsibility of the financial department. In the 1980s this trend has resulted from Medicare's reimbursement by Diagnostic Related Group. The rationale for placing medical records under finance is the fact that the Medical Records coding function has a direct impact on the institution's revenue stream. It is therefore important for the CFO to have increased communication with and control over the medical records department. This can easily be accomplished by having medical records report to finance.

THE FUNDAMENTALS OF FINANCE

The fundamentals of finance are rooted in basic accounting principles. The first two are the concepts of assets and liabilities. All businesses have assets and liabilities. An *asset* is any tangible or intangible property owned by an institution or individual. Examples include cash, accounts receivable, plant, equipment, and inventory. *Cash* is the most liquid asset available. The term *liquidity* is measured by the time it takes to convert an asset into cash to purchase something else. *Accounts receivable* are monies that will be received by the institution some time in the future. In the case of a health care institution, accounts receivable are usually for services currently rendered to a patient. *Inventory* is the actual stock on hand that the institution owns and is waiting to use in delivering future health care services.

Liabilities, on the other hand, are debts that an institution owes to other businesses. Examples include accounts payable, notes payable, bonds payable, and mortgages payable. *Accounts payable* are records of short-term debt that the institution owes a seller. An individual's Mastercard or VISA charge account are examples of an account payable. *Notes payable* are records of money owed by the institution to a seller for a loan for a period of 1 to 10 years. *Bonds payable* are records of loans made for more than 10 years that are owed by the institution. *Mortgages payable* is the record of money owed for the mortgage on the institution's property. *Wages payable* is the cash owed to employees for services received by the institution. Wages payable are frequently recorded under the heading *accrued liabilities.*

The third fundamental accounting principle is *owner's equity, fund balance,* or *net worth.* The most basic financial equation for a business can be shown as follows:

BASIC FINANCIAL EQUATION[3]

Assets = liabilities + owner's equity or net worth

In the private sector, the term owner's equity is used—this is the money the shareholders would divide if the company were to be liquidated. For example, if a for-profit hospital made the decision to go out of business, it would pay off all of its liabilities with its assets and then divide the remaining assets or owner's equity among its shareholders.

EXAMPLE

$$
\begin{array}{lr}
\text{Assets} & = \$1,000,000 \\
\text{Liabilities} & = -800,000 \\
\hline
\text{Owner's equity} & = \$\ 200,000
\end{array}
$$

$$
\frac{\text{Owner's equity}}{\text{Shares of stock}} = \frac{\$200,000}{100,000} = \$2 \text{ per share of stock}
$$

After paying off all its liabilities, this institution has $200,000 worth of assets or owner's equity remaining. This money would be divided among the shareholders by paying them $2 for each share of stock held.

After paying off all its liabilities, this institution has $200,000 worth of assets or owner's equity remaining. This money would be divided among the shareholders by paying them $2 for each share of stock held.

In the not-for-profit sector there are no shareholders. Therefore, the money that the institution accumulates from one year to another as a result of efficient operations and investing is called net worth or fund balance. *Net worth* is the difference between assets and liabilities, or what the organization is worth after all its liabilities are paid. The term *fund balance* is used by some institutions to show the excess funds they possess.

EXAMPLE

If a not-for-profit hospital has assets that total $5 million and liabilities that total $4 million, the health care organization has a net worth of $1 million dollars.

$$
\begin{array}{c}
\text{Assets} \ = \ \text{liabilities} \ + \ \text{net worth} \\
\$5 \text{ million} = \$4 \text{ million} + \$1 \text{ million}
\end{array}
$$

ACCOUNTING RECORDS

Accounting records of a business or institution are usually contained in a *general journal, general ledger,* and various *special journals* or *special ledgers.* The *general journal* is the book in which raw data is entered. Recorded information includes the date of the transaction, the affected accounts, and the magnitude and the direction of the change of the accounts. As discussed earlier, the fundamental accounting equation is written as follows:

$$\text{Assets} = \text{liabilities} + \text{owner's equity}$$

Since this equation must be kept in balance at all times, any transaction must maintain that balance. Therefore, any transaction must have at least two entries. For example, any increase in assets must be accompanied by an increase in liabilities and/or owner's equity, or any decrease in assets has an accompanying decrease in liabilities and/or owner's equity.

The double-entry accounting system has been devised to keep the relationship in constant balance. *Debits* are accounting entries that are recorded in a left-hand column, and *credits* are the entries that are recorded in a right-hand column. Debit entries must always equal credit entries.

$$\text{Debits} = \text{credits}$$

This recording mechanism is based on the fact that credits always increase owner's equity, which is located on the right-hand side of the ledger. All other increases and decreases can be documented based on the side of the equation (assets = liabilities + owner's equity) on which the account belongs.

SAMPLE PAGE OF GENERAL LEDGER

Date	Account	Debit	Credit
Jan. 2	Accounts payable	$20,000	
	Cash		$20,000
Jan. 3	Cash	1,000	
	Patient accounts receivable		1,000

This sample page of an institution's general ledger shows an entry on January 2 that represents a debit to accounts payable and a credit to cash in the sum of $20,000. This represents a payment by check of $20,000 to a medical supply company for supplies received. The debit of $20,000 to the accounts payable account represents a decrease in that account that results from payment of a bill. The corresponding credit to the cash account shows that the cash account was also decreased by issuing the check for $20,000.

The January 3 entry reflects a debit or decrease of $1,000 in patient accounts receivable and a credit or increase of $1,000 in the cash account. These entries reflect an increase of $1,000 in the institution's cash account because a patient paid $1,000 on his bill or accounts receivable account. Because of the $1,000 payment, the institution's total accounts receivable were reduced by $1,000.

Debits increase accounts to the left of the equal sign in the fundamental accounting equation (assets = liabilities + owner's equity) and credits increase accounts to the right of the equal sign. Conversely credits decrease accounts on the left side of the equation and debits decrease accounts on the right hand side.[4]

General Ledger

The general ledger summarizes the information from the general journal to show the balance in each account.

SAMPLE PAGE OF GENERAL LEDGER

Date	Debits	Credits	Balance
Jan. 1	$100,000		$100,000
Jan. 2		$20,000	80,000
Jan. 3	1,000		81,000
Jan. 4		2,000	79,000

Subsidiary Ledgers

Subsidiary ledgers are specialty ledgers that are utilized to record greater detail for specific accounts on the general ledger. In an acute care institution, a typical subsidiary ledger is created for accounts receivable. When credit is extended to patients in exchange for health care services, each patient's account receivable needs to be recorded as an individual account.

SAMPLE PATIENT ACCOUNT RECEIVABLE

Date	Debits	Credits	Balance
Jan. 1	$5,000		$5,000
Jan. 15		$2,000	3,000
Feb. 1		3,000	0

This sample subsidiary ledger documents that an account receivable for a patient was created on January 1. On January

15 and February 1 the patient made payments of $2,000 and $3,000, respectively, resulting in a bill paid in full.

There are two basic methods of accounting: *cash basis accounting* and *accrual basis accounting*. In *cash basis accounting,* revenue and expenses are recorded when they are actually collected or paid. In *accrual basis accounting,* revenue is recorded when the service is delivered, regardless of when the actual money is received. Expenses are also recorded when they occur, regardless of when actual payment is made. In this latter method of accounting, the organization is always aware of its current financial situation.

The Balance Sheet

The balance sheet is a financial document that shows the fiscal position of an organization on a particular date, by outlining what it owns and what it owes (*i.e.,* its assets and liabilities) at that point in time. As previously mentioned, assets equal liabilities plus net worth. A balance sheet can display assets and liabilities for a specific date, as well as for a number of different dates for comparison. When more than one set of assets and liabilities are compared, the result is called a *consolidated balance sheet.*[3]

The balance sheet is divided into two parts that are displayed either horizontally or vertically. Assets appear on the left side or on the top of the report. Liabilities and net worth appear on the right side or the bottom of the report. Both components of the balance sheet are always in balance or equal one another. Table 2-1 shows a very simplified balance sheet for a not-for-profit institution.

The figures on a balance sheet may drop the last group of 000's. This is noted under the title of the balance sheet by the notation *in 000's*. The balance sheet will be surveyed item by item, with definitions, methods for identification, calculation, and significance of each item included.

CURRENT ASSETS

Current assets are defined as assets that can be turned into cash within a year of the date on the balance sheet. Assets that are easily converted into cash are called *liquid assets*. The more quickly an asset can be turned into cash, the more liquid it is. Examples of current assets include cash, accounts receivable,

Table 2-1   Balance Sheet—Current Assets

	19 × 2	*19 × 1*
Current Assets		
Cash		
Checking	$ 375,000	$ 400,000
Savings	25,000	50,000
Investments	100,000	300,000
Accounts receivable		
Patient revenues	$7,000,000	$5,400,000
Less:		
Bad debts	400,000	350,000
Charitable allowances	50,000	50,000
Contractual allowances	600,000	400,000
Inventory	250,000	180,000
TOTAL CURRENT ASSETS	$6,700,000	$5,530,000

and inventories. Theoretically, they can all be converted into cash within a year.

The first component of current assets on the balance sheet is cash. Cash includes assets in checking and savings accounts as well as investments in short-term marketable securities. *Marketable securities* are short-term investments of idle or excess cash that may not be needed immediately. This cash is invested in securities such as money market funds or 30- to 90-day certificates of deposit, to earn higher interest.

EXAMPLE

Current Assets	19 × 2	19 × 1
Cash:		
Checking	$375,000	$400,000
Savings	25,000	50,000
Investments	100,000	300,000

The second major current asset is accounts receivable.

EXAMPLE

Accounts Receivable	19 × 2	19 × 1
Patients	$7,000,000	$5,400,000
Less:		
Bad debt allowance	400,000	350,000
Charitable allowances	50,000	50,000
Contractual allowances	600,000	400,000
	$5,950,000	$4,600,000

Accounts receivable are assets of the institution that will be paid by the client or patient some time in the future. When an organization extends credit to a patient, it automatically creates an account receivable. It is actually an IOU that will be received by the health care institution at some future time. Large amounts of institutional resources tied up in accounts receivable hinder the institution's ability to pay its liabilities and do other things.

Accounts receivable appear on both the balance sheet and the income statement. On the balance sheet, the first line item of accounts receivable is patient revenue outstanding on that particular date. The institution's goal is to collect all of these revenues. However, because of bad debts and contractual allowances, not all accounts receivable are collected. *Bad debts* are the revenues the institution will never collect because of patients that do not pay their bills.

On the sample balance sheet, the institution experienced $400,000 of bad debt in 19 × 2, that is, it delivered $400,000 worth of care for which it will never be reimbursed. *Charitable allowances* is the amount of revenue the institution budgets for free and/or charitable care. All health care institutions plan for providing a certain amount of charitable care that they, in turn, write off. In the past, many government grant programs were awarded to hospitals based on an institution's ability to document a certain dollar amount of free care delivered to the community.

The third reduction to patient revenues, *contractual allowances,* results from the difference between the revenues actually reimbursed to the hospital, and the actual charges issued by the institution. Contractual allowances are the discounts given to third-party payors through negotiation or contracting. As a third-party payor, Medicare has stipulated the DRG payments it is willing to reimburse hospitals for specific conditions.

When hospital charges are greater than the Medicare DRG payment or the third-party contract rate, the hospital reduces it gross patient revenues by subtracting the contractual allowance. On the other hand, there are instances where the DRG rate is greater than the hospital charges. In the latter case, the contractual allowance is an addition to patient revenues.

Hospital charges are the hospital's costs plus a mark-up factor. Hospital *costs*, on the other hand, are the actual amount of money that is required to produce a product or deliver a patient care service.

EXAMPLE

Cost = actual money required to deliver patient care services
Charge = cost plus mark-up factor

If an institution billed for charges of $7,750,000 and was reimbursed $7,150,000 by Medicare and third-party payors for those patients, the institution experienced contractual allowances totaling $600,000.

SAMPLE CALCULATIONS

Actual hospital charges −	Medicare + third-party reimbursement		contractual allowance or loss
$7,750,000	−	$7,150,000	=	($600,000)

As discussed earlier, Medicare's prospective DRG reimbursement rates and third-party per diem contract rates fall short of the institution's retrospective charges, resulting in contractual allowances. These contractual allowances are actual reductions to the institution's revenue stream. The reductions of bad debt, and charitable and contractual allowances are subtracted from the billed accounts receivable in 19×2 to total $5,950,000, which is expected to be collected in the future.

It is important to note that on the balance sheet the accounts receivable that appear are accounts billed to the date of the balance sheet. Bad debt and contractual allowances that appear on the balance sheet are confirmed reductions that actually have been written off. Once the reduction appears on the balance sheet, it is assumed that there will be no future opportunity to recover these revenues. On the other hand, the resources that appear in accounts receivable on the same statement could also contain future bad debts and contractual allowances.

The final component of current assets is inventories. *Inventory* is the actual stock on hand that the institution owns and is storing for use in delivering health care services in the future. Inventories are considered current assets because they can be converted into cash fairly easily. Inventories appear on both the balance sheet and the income statement.

In a health care institution, inventories are composed of medical and non-medical supplies, drugs, food, cleaned linen, and so on. Supplies in inventory are usually valued on the balance sheet by actual cost or market price, whichever is lower. This is done to yield a conservative figure for inventories. Inventories are usually valued conservatively to account for factors such as deterioration and obsolescence.

EXAMPLE

	19 × 2	19 × 1
Inventories	$250,000	$180,000

Specific methods for valuing inventories and efficient management of inventories are discussed in more detail later in this chapter.

In summary, current assets that appear on a hospital's balance sheet include the following:

- Cash
- Accounts receivable
- Inventories

Reductions to current assets include the following:

- Allowances for bad debt
- Charitable allowances
- Contractual allowances

Putting all these factors together, current assets on the balance sheet add up to *total current assets*. For an example, see Table 2-1.

FIXED ASSETS

Fixed assets are long-term assets that are more commonly referred to as property, plant or buildings, and equipment. Fixed assets have value that can be converted into cash in the long term. Examples of fixed assets for a health care institution include the following:

Land: This is the property owned by the institution. It can include the land on which the primary facility is located, as well as land owned by the institution for future development and/or speculation.

Buildings: Buildings include the hospital, doctors' office buildings, outpatient clinics, and skilled nursing facilities that the institution owns.

Equipment: Equipment includes CT scanners, x-ray machines, surgical and laboratory equipment, and so on.

Construction: Most institutions are continuously undergoing improvement or replacement construction programs. Completed portions of the construction programs appear here under fixed assets (Table 2-2).

DEPRECIATION

Depreciation is a reduction in the value of fixed assets or buildings and equipment, based on the concept that they loose some of their usefulness and utility over time. When a piece of equipment such as a CT scanner is used over a period of time, it begins to wear out or may even become obsolete. Depreciation is the way in which the institution shows that the CT scanner "wears out" in financial terms on the balance sheet. Depreciation is not an actual loss or expense to the institution in the respect that money actually goes out of the institution. It is, however, an expense on the balance sheet in an accounting sense that represents the symbolic cost of using a piece of equipment for a period of time and "using up" some of its value. (Specific methods for calculating depreciation will be discussed later in this chapter.) Depreciation is then subtracted from

Table 2-2   Balance Sheet—Fixed Assets

	19 × 2	19 × 1
Fixed Assets		
Land	$ 4,500,000	$ 4,500,000
Buildings	15,800,000	15,000,000
Equipment	5,500,000	3,000,000
Construction in progress	2,500,000	800,000
Subtotal	28,300,000	23,300,000
Less: Depreciation	$ 4,800,000	$ 3,700,000
Net fixed assets	$23,500,000	$19,600,000
TOTAL ASSETS	$30,200,000	$25,130,000

fixed assets to determine *net fixed assets.* Current assets are added to net fixed assets to create total assets.

LIABILITIES AND NET WORTH

The second part of the balance sheet consists of liabilities and net worth, as discussed earlier in the chapter.The liabilities and net worth of the sample institution are shown in Table 2-3.

Current Liabilities. Liabilities are debts of the institution that are classified by their maturity. Maturity refers to the age of a liability or when it will be repaid by the institution. Current liabilities are paid within 12 months, whereas long-term debts are paid after a 12-month period. Specific current liabilities appearing on a hospital's balance sheet include the following:

> *Accounts payable* include unpaid balances owed to drug distributors, medical supply companies, non-medical supply companies, food distributors, and so on. These bills or debts are usually paid within 30, 60, or 90 days.

> *Notes payable* are short-term promissory notes owed to a bank or other lending agency. They are usually paid within a year.

> *Accrued liabilities* or *accrued expenses payable* include any short-term expenses such as insurance premiums, attorneys' fees, employees' wages and salaries, pensions, and medical fees that have not been paid as of the date on the balance sheet. These are referred to as *wages payable* in some institutions.

Table 2-3   Balance Sheet — Liabilities and Net Worth

	19 × 2	*19 × 1*
Current Liabilities		
Accounts payable	$ 3,500,000	$ 2,500,000
Notes payable	300,000	450,000
Wages payable (accrued liabilities)	100,000	90,000
Current portion of term debt	200,000	50,000
TOTAL CURRENT LIABILITIES	$ 4,100,000	$ 3,090,000
Long-Term Liabilities		
Bonds payable	$21,000,000	$20,000,000
Mortgage payable	500,000	650,000
TOTAL LIABILITIES	$25,600,000	$23,740,000
Net Worth	$ 4,600,000	$ 1,390,000
Total Liabilities and Net Worth	$30,200,000	$25,130,000

Federal income taxes appear under current liabilities for the for-profit health care institutions because they are due on an annual basis.

Long-Term Liabilities. Long-term liabilities are debts of the institution that are due more than a year after the date on the balance sheet. Examples of long-term liabilities that appear on a health care balance sheet include the following:

Bonds payable are formal promissory notes issued by the institution in exchange for cash. The promissory note is held by the bondholder who paid cash for it. The health care institution, in turn, agrees to pay the bondholder annual interest on the debt, and the principal in a certain number of years (*e.g.*, 5 to 10 years). The interest on the bond is usually paid on a semiannual basis and appears on the income statement as an expense for the institution called *interest expense*.

Interest expense is paid by the institution to the bondholder for the use of the bondholder's money.

Mortgages payable is long-term debt on the institution's building. On the balance sheet, mortgage payable represents the balance the institution owes on its mortgage.

The example compares the institution's long-term liabilities for 2 specific years. Bonds payable increased from $20,000,000 to $21,000,000 from the first year to the second year. This means that the institution issued additional bonds between the 2 years resulting in an actual increase in the bonds that will need to be paid back by the institution. Because the institution has an increase in outstanding bonds, it is also possible to anticipate that the institution will be paying higher interest expenses in the second year because of the greater amount of outstanding bonds.

The example also reflects the fact that the institution reduced its mortgage payable liability by $150,000 from the first year to the second as a result of payment of that debt.

Net Worth. As previously outlined, assets − liabilities = net worth. Net worth is sometimes referred to as *fund balance* on a not-for-profit institution's balance sheet and *owner's equity* or *stockholder's equity* on the balance sheet of a for-profit institution. *Net worth* is the worth or value of the institution after paying all its debts or liabilities. When the term *net worth* is used on the balance sheet, all excess funds are included under a one-line item like this:

EXAMPLE

	19 × 2	19 × 1
Net worth	$4,600,000	$1,390,000

When *fund balance* is used on the balance sheet, it is common to include the factors shown in Table 2-4.

This example shows that the institution experienced an $800,000 loss in the past year and a $2,300,000 profit in the current year. *Note:* Whenever an entry is enclosed in parentheses, an unfavorable condition is present.

In the for-profit health care institutions, excess funds or assets are called *owner's equity* or *stockholder's equity*. In the private sector, this equity is the source of the funds that are distributed to stockholders in the form of dividends. Dividends are a percentage of the profits that the organization yields and that are, in turn, shared with the stockholders. Dividends are first paid to stockholders that hold preferred stock, and then dividends are paid to common stockholders.

The institution may choose to retain some of its profits within the institution for future growth and investment. This is reflected in the line item *retained earnings* on the balance sheet. Retained earnings are the profits the institution chooses to retain in the organization for future growth, expansion, and investments, rather than divide among stockholders as dividends. Owner's equity appears on the balance sheet as shown in Table 2-5.

When the final component of net worth, fund balance, or

Table 2-4   Balance Sheet—Fund Balance

	19 × 2	19 × 1
Fund Balance		
Fund balance at beginning of year	$2,300,000	$2,190,000
Current year net income (loss)	2,300,000	(800,000)
TOTAL FUND BALANCE	$4,600,000	$1,390,000

Table 2-5   Balance Sheet — Owner's Equity

	19 X 2	19 X 1
Owner's Equity		
Preferred stock	$ 700,000	$ 190,000
Common stock	2,000,000	800,000
Retained earnings	1,900,000	400,000
TOTAL OWNER'S EQUITY	$4,600,000	$1,390,000

owner's equity is added to total liabilities, the balance sheet is completed. By putting all the components together, the balance sheet is complete (see Table 2-6).

Table 2-6   Balance Sheet 19 X 2

	19 X 2	19 X 1
Current Assets		
Cash	$ 500,000	$ 750,000
Accounts receivable		
Patient Revenues	7,000,000	5,400,000
Less:		
Bad debts	400,000	350,000
Charitable allowances	50,000	50,000
Contractual allowances	600,000	400,000
Inventory	250,000	180,000
TOTAL CURRENT ASSETS	$ 6,700,000	$ 5,530,000
Fixed Assets		
Land	$ 4,500,000	$ 4,500,000
Buildings (plant)	15,800,000	15,000,000
Equipment	5,500,000	3,000,000
Construction in progress	2,500,000	800,000
	$28,300,000	$23,300,000
Less: Depreciation	4,800,000	3,700,000
NET FIXED ASSETS	$23,500,000	$19,600,000
TOTAL ASSETS	$30,200,000	$25,130,000
Current Liabilities		
Accounts payable	$ 3,500,000	$ 2,500,000
Notes payable	300,000	450,000
Accrued liabilities	100,000	90,000
Current portion of long-term debt	200,000	50,000
TOTAL CURRENT LIABILITIES	$ 4,100,000	$ 3,090,000
Long-Term Liabilities		
Bonds payable	$21,000,000	$20,000,000
Mortgage payable	500,000	650,000
Net Worth	4,600,000	1,390,000
Total Liabilities and Net Worth	$30,200,000	$25,130,000

Income Statement

The second major financial report of importance is the income statement, which can serve as a valuable tool in anticipating the future performance and/or success of an organization. It exhibits revenue and expenses for one or more years. An income statement that includes more than 1 year's data is called a consolidated income statement, and is mainly used to compare the company's performance over a couple of years.

The *income statement* is a record of the money or revenue coming into the organization for services rendered, and the money that leaves the organization because of expenses. Revenue can be subdivided into operating revenue and non-operating revenue. *Operating revenue* is generated by the sale of the institution's goods and/or services (*e.g.*, emergency care services in an acute care institution). *Non-operating revenue,* on the other hand, is revenue obtained from sources other than the institution's major business. Interest income from an organization's securities is an example of non-operating revenue.

Expenses are divided into operating and non-operating expenses. *Operating expenses* include the cost of goods or products sold, overhead expenses such as wages and salaries, rent, supplies, mortgage payments, and depreciation. *Non-operating expenses* include interest expenses and taxes in the for-profit sector. These various sources of revenues and kinds of expenses will be dealt with individually, as actually experienced in a health care institution.

The common financial term *"the bottom line"* is the result of subtracting *total operating expenses* from net patient revenues. Another term for "bottom line" is *net income from operations.*

A hospital's operating margin can be calculated by dividing net income from operations by net revenue from patients. *Operating margin* is the percentage of profit that the organization makes from the operations of its major business. *Profit* is basically the difference between net expenses and net revenue. In the for-profit sector, the profit or difference between expenses and revenue are further reduced by taxes.

REVENUE

The organization's most important source of revenue appears on the first line of the income statement. The major revenue source for a health care organization is the delivery of health care services to patients.

Health care institutions care for many different individuals; however, the services they provide are paid for by relatively few sources. These payors include the following:

1. Third-party insurance companies
2. Federal Medicare program
3. State Medicaid Programs
4. Individuals
5. Capitated health maintenance organizations

Third-party payors include all of the above payors except the individual . The hospital and the patient constitute the first "two parties" in the delivery of health care services. Therefore, a third party is any agent with whom the patient contracts to pay part or all of his health care bills.

Third-party payors are the major source of revenue for most hospitals. An institution's third-party payor mix has a strong impact on its financial health and stability. Medicare is the federal government's health insurance for individuals over the age of 65 and/or who are disabled. As previously mentioned, the program is undergoing significant changes and reductions in the mid-1980s. Medicaid is the state health insurance for the poor. Capitated health maintenance organizations (HMOs) charge employers or individuals a per head rate to keep their enrollees healthy. When enrollees must be hospitalized, the cost of that hospitalization reduces the profits of the HMO. When enrollees are cared for without requiring hospitalization, the HMO retains more of its resources.

On most health care income statements, the first line on the income statement is called revenue from routine patient services. Revenue from ancillary services usually appears on the second revenue line, and is revenue that is received from the delivery of respiratory therapy, EKG, radiology services, and so on. Total gross patient revenues is the amount of money that would be received by the organization if all bills were paid as submitted. This is rarely the case, however. In a health care setting, there are various factors that reduce the amount of revenue that the institution actually collects. These factors include the following:

1. Allowances for bad debt
2. Charitable allowances
3. Contractural allowances

These allowances and reductions are subtracted from gross patient revenues to form net patient revenues (Table 2-7). Net patient revenues are the funds the institution receives after subtracting these reductions and allowances for bad debt, charity, and contracts.

OPERATING EXPENSES

Operating expenses include all the institution's expenses to maintain the ongoing and routine operations of the organization. In the health care industry, operating expenses include the following:

Salaries are the wages paid to employees of the institution. Salary expenses can be divided into direct and indirect salary expenses. Direct salary expenses reflect direct nursing care, whereas indirect salary expenses account for management salaries.

Employee benefits include employee health insurance, holiday pay, vacation pay, and the sick pay that the institution pays employees.

Medical supplies include items such as soap, lotion, tissues, Chux, Foley catheters, and so on.

Non-medical supplies include supplies such as forms, stationery, paper, paper clips, and so on.

Medical fees and *commissions* include payments to physicians for administrative or clinical services.

Purchased services is a line of operational expenses that

Table 2-7 Income Statement—Revenue

	19 × 2	19 × 1
Gross patient (revenue)	$37,000,000	$30,400,000
Less:		
Bad debt	700,000	550,000
Charity	150,000	100,000
Contractual allowances	4,600,000	2,400,000
	$ 5,450,000	$ 3,050,000
NET PATIENT REVENUE	$31,550,000	$27,350,000

usually includes fees for occasionally utilized services, and consultant and management fees.

Maintenance and *utilities* expenses represent the cost of maintaining the institution's plant and equipment.

Professional liability insurance is the institution's cost for liability insurance.

Financing costs are the expenses an institution experiences in borrowing money to replace and/or improve its plant and equipment.

Depreciation is the expense on the financial statements that represents the loss in value of an asset over time.

DEPRECIATION

Depreciation is classified as a general operational expense, and is defined as the decline in the useful value of an asset because of wear and tear. There are various methods of depreciating an asset.

Table 2-8   Income Statement 19 × 2

	19 × 2	*19 × 1*
Gross Patient Revenues		
Routine patient services	$12,000,000	$10,000,000
Ancillary services	25,000,000	20,400,000
TOTAL GROSS PATIENT REVENUE	$37,000,000	$30,400,000
Deductions from Revenues		
Provision for bad debt	700,000	550,000
Charitable allowance	150,000	100,000
Contractual allowance	4,600,000	2,400,000
TOTAL DEDUCTIONS	$ 5,450,000	3,050,000
NET REVENUES FROM PATIENTS	$31,550,000	$27,350,000
Operating Expenses		
Salaries	$14,500,000	$11,000,000
Employee benefits	1,200,000	900,000
Medical supplies	2,500,000	2,800,000
Non-medical supplies	1,400,000	1,900,000
Medical fees and commissions	2,200,000	1,950,000
Purchased services	900,000	750,000
Maintenance and utilities	1,500,000	1,350,000
Professional liability	350,000	300,000
Financing costs	1,200,000	1,010,000
Depreciation	900,000	700,000
TOTAL OPERATING EXPENSES	$26,650,000	$22,660,000
Net Income from Operations	$ 4,900,000	4,690,000
Operating Margin	15.5%	17.1%

Because of its unique nature, depreciation is included on a separate line on the income statement. Depreciation is an accounting expense that leaves the organization via the income statement. It is not a real money expense, however. Depreciation is an expense to the organization that shows some of an asset has been "used up" over the past year. The depreciation expense allows the organization to show that a reduction of an asset has occurred, based on its use over a year's period of time. If depreciation were not included, expenses would be understated and profits would be overstated. Depreciation supports the concept that capital assets and/or equipment use themselves up and lose some of their utility. Depreciation is the method of stating this concept in financial terms on the financial statements.

Assets must have a useful life exceeding 1 year to qualify for a depreciation deduction. Only business assets can be depreciated—personal assets cannot be depreciated. Land is never depreciated because it is believed to possess an indefinite useful life. The useful life of an asset is defined as the period of time it is useful to the owner. It may be that an asset such as a CT scanner could be functional for a period of 10 years, but be obsolete after 5 years. The CT scanner could be depreciated, in this case over a period of 5 years. The Internal Revenue Service has comprehensive guidelines for the appropriate depreciation of assets.

There are two different ways to depreciate an asset: straight-line depreciation and accelerated depreciation.

Straight-Line Depreciation. The straight-line method of depreciation subtracts the salvage value of the asset from the purchase price, and then divides the remainder by the number of useful years of life for the asset.[5] For example, if a CT scanner is purchased for $800,000 and can be salvaged in 5 years (when it becomes obsolete) for $50,000, annual depreciation can be calculated in this manner:

CALCULATIONS FOR STRAIGHT-LINE DEPRECIATION

Initial cost − salvage value ÷ years depreciated = annual depreciation
$800,000 − $50,000 = $750,000 ÷ 5 years = $150,000
$150,000 = the annual depreciation deduction for the institution

---

The health care institution can deduct $150,000 for depreciation annually for the CT scanner for each of the 5 years. They can enter $150,000 in depreciation expense on the income statement and the balance sheet for the CT scanner each year.

At the end of each year, the CT scanner would be valued on the balance sheet as follows:

EXAMPLE

Year	Depreciation Deducted on Income Statement	Value of CT Scanner on Balance Sheet
19 × 1	$150,000	$650,000
19 × 2	$150,000	$500,000
19 × 3	$150,000	$350,000
19 × 4	$150,000	$200,000
19 × 5	$150,000	$ 50,000

Double-Declining-Balance Method. The double-declining-balance method is an accelerated depreciation method that is also called the 200% declining balance method. This method can be used for new tangible property having a useful life of at least 3 years. The double-declining-balance method depreciates an asset twice as fast as straight-line depreciation, but only to the point of the salvage value level.[5] According to the straight-line depreciation method, the asset was depreciated at a rate of 20% annually. (Twenty percent = one-fifth of the useful life of the scanner.) The double-declining-balance method depreciates an asset twice as fast as straight-line depreciation, and so the scanner would be depreciated at an annual rate of 40%. In the double-declining-balance method, the salvage value is not deducted from the purchase price in the first year, as in straight-line depreciation. The asset is depreciated down to the salvage value, or $50,000. The following calculations show how the same CT scanner would be depreciated by the double-declining-balance method:

EXAMPLE: DOUBLE-DECLINING-BALANCE METHOD

Year	Depreciation on Income Statement	Book Value on Balance Sheet
19 × 1	$800,000 × .40 = $320,000	$480,000
19 × 2	$480,000 × .40 = $152,000	$328,000
19 × 3	$328,000 × .40 = $131,200	$196,800
19 × 4	$196,800 × .40 = $ 78,720	$118,080
19 × 5	$118,080 × .40 = $ 47,232	$ 70,848

After depreciation is calculated, total operating expenses are subtracted from net revenues from patients to form net income from operations. The institution's operating margin can be calculated by dividing net income from operations by net revenue from patients.

CALCULATION OF OPERATING MARGIN

$$\frac{\text{Net income from operations}}{\text{Net revenues from patients}} = \frac{\$4,900,000}{\$31,550,000} = 15.5\%$$

Operating margin = 15.5%

See Table 2-8 for the completed income statement.

MANAGEMENT OF ACCOUNTS RECEIVABLE

As outlined previously, when any organization extends credit to a client, an account receivable is created. That account or IOU will be received by the hospital at some future time. A major concern for the hospital is *when* in the future the account will be paid by the patient. This is important because of the time-value concept of money and the institution's cash-flow position.

The time-value concept of money acknowledges that when a company has an account receivable rather than the cash, it loses the interest income the cash could generate if the institution invested it. The time-value concept of money is also called the *opportunity cost*. If a hospital has an account receivable rather than cash, the hospital lacks the ability to take advantage of various opportunities because of a lack of cash. The hospital has paid an opportunity cost or loss as a result of having the account receivable rather than cash.

EXAMPLE

Accounts receivable	= $100,000
Age = 90 days	
Current interest rate for	= 10%
3-month certificate of deposits	

Accounts receivable × current interest rate = interest income

$100,000	×	.10	=	$10,000
Institution's lost interest income or			=	$10,000
opportunity cost				

The second important factor of accounts receivable is their impact on the institution's cash flow.

Cash flow is the amount of cash that an organization has coming in at any point in time. As mentioned previously, cash is the most liquid of all assets and is necessary for the organization to pay its current debts or liabilities in a timely manner. When the institution has many accounts receivable outstanding for excessive periods, it does not have use of that cash to pay its current debts. Employees' salaries are probably the most important current debt a hospital must be able to pay in a timely manner.

In the current economic environment of health care, patient accounts receivable are more difficult to collect, and it is very important that they be managed properly if the health care institution is to survive and prosper. Effective management of accounts receivable involves a basic understanding of the accounts receivable cycle and the effects of varying credit policies on the collection of those receivables.

Accounts Receivable Cycle

The cycle of accounts receivable begins when an institution delivers health care services to a patient for credit. This constitutes the *creation* of an account receivable. When cash is received for the health care services that are rendered, this is termed *collection*. Management of accounts receivable includes estimating which accounts may not be collected in full (adjusted accounts) and which accounts may not be collected at all (write-off accounts).

Whenever an institution accepts credit for services rendered, it must realize that a certain percentage of those accounts will not be collected in full, and some will never be collected. Generally, as the length of time for collecting an account receivable increases, the greater the chance it will never be collected and will have to be written off. Institutions acknowledge these facts fiscally by including a specific figure in the budget for allowances or provisions for bad debts. The budgeted and actual figures for bad debts that are written off are then subtracted from gross patient revenues (see Table 2-9).

In this budget example, the first deduction, or $3,700,000, was budgeted for bad debts or accounts that would never be collected. $4,000,000 of accounts receivable was actually written

Table 2-9   Statement of Revenues and Expenses ($ in 000's)

	Actual	Budget	Var.
Total gross patient revenue	$7,000	$9,600	(2,600)
Deductions from revenue			
Provisions for bad debt	4,000	3,700	(300)
Charitable allowances	50	90	40
Contractual allowances	600	400	(200)
Total deductions	4,650	4,190	(460)
Net revenue from patients	2,350	5,410	(3,060)

off, resulting in a variance of $300,000 in excess of what was budgeted.

The second line deduction from gross patient revenues is charitable allowances. This is the amount the institution budgeted and actually wrote off for services rendered to the poor or medically indigent adults (MIAs). The institution budgeted $90,000 in charitable allowances, but experienced only $50,000 of charitable services delivered without reimbursement.

The third and final line of deductions reflects contractual allowances or the difference between charges for health care services and reimbursement for those services. In the 1980s, this line item reflects the following allowances or losses:

1. The difference between hospital charges and Medicare's flat DRG reimbursement rate

EXAMPLE: NINE-DAY LENGTH OF STAY FOR A MYOCARDIAL INFARCTION PATIENT

Calculations:

Hospital charges for	−	DRG reimbursement	=	Contractual
acute MI patient		for DRG #122		allowance (loss)
$9,500	−	$5,300	=	($4,200)

2. The difference between hospital charges for health care services and third-party per diem contract rate multiplied by the patient's length of stay

EXAMPLE

Calculations:

Charges for services	−	(per diem contract rate)	=	Contractual
for acute MI		× length of stay		allowance (loss)
$9,500	−	($500 × 9 = $4,500)	=	($5,000)

In this example, the institution has a contract with a third-party payor for all its services for $500 per day. The institution is reimbursed $500 per day times the patient's length of stay, or $500 × 9 days = $4500. The charges for services rendered to the acute MI patient actually totaled $9,500. The contractual allowances or losses on this patient equal $5,000.

The total deductions are subtracted from gross patient revenues to equal *net revenue from patients*. It is very important for institutions to acknowledge that these deductions do exist and to budget accurately for them. If these deductions are underestimated, they will significantly erode or reduce the actual bottom line because net revenues will be overstated on the budget figures.

This discussion of reductions and allowances to revenue shows that appropriate management of accounts receivable is very important to the fiscal health of the organization. The most important aspect of managing accounts receivable is the institution's credit policy. If an institution would insist on receiving cash for all services prior to rendering the service, it would never need to worry about the losses associated with accounts receivable. However, few health care consumers are capable of paying cash up front for hospital services. The institution would experience a low census and a low demand for services, because of the minority of individuals capable of paying cash before services are rendered.

Therefore, most organizations and literally all health care institutions do accept varying levels of credit. They trade increased volume of patients for an increased risk of experiencing some losses or bad debt. When identifying an appropriate credit policy for an institution, two factors should be considered:

1. The effect a specific credit policy has on patient demand for services and the institution's cash flow
2. The costs associated with creating and maintaining accounts receivable

Credit policies may range from very permissive to very restrictive, based on the institution's leadership, fiscal health, demand, and the costs to manage accounts receivable.

An account receivable undergoes an "aging" process as it

moves from creation to payment or write-off.[5] The "aging" process and appropriate interventions utilized to receive payments on the account are usually determined by the chief financial officer (CFO) of the institution. Table 2-10 shows the "aging" process of an account receivable with specific interventions that can be utilized by the institution to collect the monies.

In the private sector, interest penalties are charged on accounts that are delinquent. The maximun interest penalty is fixed by law and calculated from the time the account is due to the date it is actually paid. Few health care institutions have charged interest penalties in the past, but this may be a reasonable strategy to decrease an institution's days in receivables and thereby improve its cash flow.

INVENTORY MANAGEMENT

The term *inventory* has various meanings for different businesses. In manufacturing companies, inventories include raw materials, work-in-progress, and finished goods. An example of raw materials is lumber that will be used for making furniture. In the health care setting, raw materials could include the produce, meat, and poultry in the refrigerated units that will be used for patient meals. Works-in-progress inventories are goods that are partially completed. In a manufacturing company, this could be furniture frames that have not yet been upholstered. In a hospital, work-in-progress inventories could include assembled procedure trays in central supply that have not yet been wrapped and sterilized.

Finished goods inventory are goods that require no further processing and are ready for use. In an acute health care setting, pre-mixed IV solutions are an example of finished goods inventory. Supplies account for approximately 12% to 15% of non-wage expenses in an acute care institution. Therefore,

Table 2-10   Aging of Accounts Receivable

Age	0–15 Days	15–30 Days	30–40 Days	45–60 Days	>60
Intervention	Creation of AR	First notice	Second notice	Third notice	Write-off

management of supplies or inventory involves a significant amount of the institution's capital. When inventory management and control are not appropriately carried out, large amounts of the institution's capital are tied up in inventory. When capital is tied up in this manner, the institution loses the use and availability of that capital.

Inventory management is tied to the control of supplies via an internal control mechanism, accounts payable management, and purchasing policies. Major challenges in the appropriate management of inventories in health care revolve around the unpredictable nature of the demand for health care services, as well as the life-and-death nature of some health care services. In managing inventories, it is important not to tie up excess capital in stock or inventory. On the other hand, if inventory of a particular item is used up, the institution's supply may run out. Supplies such as temporary pacemakers and endotracheal tubes may be infrequently used items, yet capable of determining life and death in certain circumstances. Because of these factors, nurses have traditionally stock-piled supplies (maintained excessive inventories) to ensure that they "never ran out." This is an important area for nurse administrators to focus on in a cost-conscious operating environment.

The cost to an organization to maintain various levels of inventory include the following specific costs:

1. *Purchasing cost* is the actual price paid to a supplier for a product. The purchasing cost of a product usually varies with the quantity ordered. The size of the quantity ordered is a significant factor in determining cost per unit and total cost of inventory maintained.

2. *Order cost* is the total administrative cost involved in the purchase of supplies. These administrative costs include evaluating various products, identifying supply specifications, soliciting and analyzing bids, and processing orders, invoices, goods, and returning goods.

3. *Carrying cost* is the cost of storing the inventory and capital funds invested in inventory.

The opportunity cost associated with inventory is calculated by identifying the highest rate of return that could be obtained if the capital invested in the inventory were invested in another way.

EXAMPLE

A critical care unit has an inventory of Swan-Ganz catheters totaling $5,000. The current rate of interest that the institution could obtain is 8%.

$$\text{Opportunity cost} = \$5,000 \times 8\% = \$400$$
$$\text{Opportunity cost} = \$400$$

This opportunity cost represents the fact that if the critical care unit would put the $5,000 in another investment, they could have made $400 in interest income. Therefore, the opportunity cost the unit is paying to maintain a $5000 Swan-Ganz inventory is $400.

The storage portion of the carrying cost includes the portion of space needed to store the actual supplies, as well allocation of overhead expenses (*e.g.*, lights and electricity, for the inventory space).

4. *Long* or *overstock costs* are the costs associated with certain supplies becoming outdated or expired and not being usable.

5. *Short* or *stock-out costs* are the costs incurred when the company runs out of a particular product and therefore loses a customer and the associated revenue. For example, if an acute care institution were to run out of Swan-Ganz catheters, a patient requiring one in the critical care unit would need to be transferred to another facility. The first institution incurs a stock-out cost that is equivalent to the revenue it lost as a result of the patient being transferred to the other facility. In addition to this stock-out cost, this situation could lead to excessive patient risk.

Methods of Valuing Inventories

There are four methods to value inventories on the balance sheet. They include (1) LIFO (last-in, first-out), (2) FIFO (first-in, first-out), (3) specific identification, and (4) weighted-average method. In LIFO, a company utilizes the replacement cost of the last unit of a good to go into inventory, as the cost of that good for the financial statements. *LIFO* values inventories at a cost that most approximates the replacement cost of the good. *Replacement cost* is the cost to replace a good at a specific point in time. Because of economic factors such as inflation and competition, the cost to replace a specific item varies over time.

While LIFO values inventories that are being sold closest to the actual replacement costs, it actually understates the remaining goods in inventories. LIFO states profits more conservatively because it matches current costs more closely with current selling prices.[6]

For example, the central supply department of a hospital maintains an adequate inventory of bedpans for patient use. An item such as a bedpan does not expire, and so the department may choose any method to deal with inventory. Let us say that bedpans are ordered on an as-needed basis, and an inventory of 100 bedpans is maintained. Because of various market influences, the central supply department has paid the following prices for bedpans over the past 6 months.

EXAMPLE

Month	Cost/Unit	Units Ordered
Jan	1.50	175
Feb	1.55	150
Mar	1.48	200
Apr	1.65	175
May	1.70	150
Jun	1.75	150

LIFO takes bedpans out of stock at the last price first and then works backwards, depending on how many bedpans are needed. As new stock is purchased, it is added to the bottom of the price list, and that is the price the next bedpans are valued at out of stock. If 150 bedpans were used in July, they would be taken out of inventory at the "last-in" price of $1.75 per bedpan. If 200 bedpans were used, 150 bedpans would leave the inventory at a price of $1.75 per bedpan, and 50 would be taken out at the next price of $1.70 per bedpan.

Therefore, the July balance sheet would value the remaining bedpan inventory as shown in Table 2-11.

Table 2-11 Calculations for Valuing Inventory Using LIFO

Month Entered Inventory	Cost/Unit		Units in Inventory		Value of Inventory
Jan	$1.50	×	175	=	$ 262.50
Feb	$1.55	×	150	=	$ 232.50
Mar	$1.48	×	200	=	$ 296.00
Apr	$1.65	×	175	=	$ 288.75
May	$1.70	×	100	=	$ 170.00
Jun	$ .75	×	0	=	0
Total inventory				=	$1,249.75

If the department used a FIFO system of valuing the inventory, the inventory value would be greater. *FIFO* is the valuing method that calls for first-in, first-out. Under FIFO, the same utilization of 200 bedpans for July would create the following inventory value shown in Table 2-12.

Specific identification is the inventory valuing method that tags each item with its actual price. When the inventory is valued, each tagged item in the inventory is added up to determine the total value of the inventory.

The *weighted average* method adds up the total costs of each item in the inventory, and divides by the number of items in the inventory. As each item is removed from the inventory, the weighted average cost of the inventory actually changes.

These various examples and sample calculations show that the institution's assets can be influenced by the specific accounting method used for valuing inventories. Inventories are valued conservatively using LIFO, and more closely resemble current or replacement costs when using FIFO.

FINANCING CAPITAL

Institutions can obtain funds from two basic sources: equity and/or debt. *Equity* is the owner's investment or the value owned in the institution. Examples of equity financing include the selling of stocks or use of the hospital's retained earnings as a source of capital.

Debt financing is a short- or long-term loan to an institution that must be repaid. Examples of debt financing include the issuing of bonds and taking out of loans from banks or other

Table 2-12   Calculations for Valuing Inventory Under FIFO

Month Purchased Inventory	Cost/Unit		Units in Inventory		Value of Inventory
Jan	$1.50	×	0	=	0
Feb	$1.55	×	125	=	$ 193.75
Mar	$1.48	×	200	=	$ 296.00
Apr	$1.65	×	175	=	$ 288.75
May	$1.70	×	150	=	$ 255.00
Jun	$1.75	×	150	=	$ 262.50
Total inventory				=	$1,296.00

lending institutions. Each one of these financing alternatives will be defined and examined individually for use by health care institutions.

Stock

Only for-profit institutions may issue stock to the public. Therefore, at the current time this financing strategy is not an alternative for not-for-profit institutions. When a for-profit institution issues stock, the funds it receives in return for the stock never has to be repaid. Once the institution has these funds, they can use them forever. The institution usually pays dividends to its stockholders based on its profits and losses. Also, as the profits of the institution grow, the value of the stock rises. The stockholder can make a profit by selling his stock to other individuals at a higher price than he paid for it. A major disadvantage of using stock to finance capital is that dividend payments are not deductible for income tax purposes.

Bond Financing

An institution finances capital through bonds by selling IOUs to individuals in exchange for cash. The process of issuing bonds is as follows:

- A hospital identifies the amount of capital it desires to finance a particular project (*e.g.*, expansion or replacement project).
- The institution applies to a bond rating agency such as Moody's or Standard & Poor's for a credit rating. The rating it achieves is based on the organization's past financial performance. The rating will determine the rate of interest it will have to pay its bondholders for the use of their money.
- The rating agency evaluates the institution's past financial performance to determine the level of risk for the bondholders' investments. The better the past financial performance, the better the rating will be and the lower will be the interest rate that the institution needs to pay bondholders for the use of their money. The most secure investments are given a rating of Aaa by Moody's and AAA by Standard and Poor's. The most common rating for a health care institution is A. Medium-grade bonds are rated down to Bbb and BBB. Medium-grade bonds involve greater risk and therefore pay a higher interest rate.

- The bonds are sold or issued in specific denominations (e.g., $5,000 for a specific period of time, such as 10 years, and at a certain interest rate, such as 9% interest.

- The institution pays interest semi-annually to the bondholders for the entire life of the bond. The interest paid the bondholders appears on the income statement as interest expense.

- At the end of the life of the bond, the institution repays the bondholder the face value of the bond, which is equal to the original loan. When the institution repays the bondholder, the money appears on the income statement as *bonds due*.

Cost of Capital/Compound Interest Effects

Access to capital is essential for the growth and expansion of any organization. There are costs associated with the acquisition and/or use of capital. These costs result from the time value concept of money. The *time value concept of money* states that a dollar today is worth more than a dollar in the future. Therefore, if an individual or institution desires to borrow money today, there is a cost to borrow that money. The cost of borrowing money or capital is the interest rate.

The cost of borrowing capital is an important factor to consider in financial decision making. This cost of capital is also called the *theory of compound interest* or the "math of finance."[7] It is essential to understand the concept of compound interest when dealing with various capital decision alternatives. All capital expenditures occur over a number of years and, therefore, include the cost of borrowing capital. This added cost is then added to the cost of the capital item. Compound interest is calculated by the following equation:

CALCULATIONS FOR COMPUTING COMPOUND INTEREST

$V_t = P_0(1 + i)^t$
V_t = final cost of capital equipment
P_0 = beginning cost of capital equipment
i = interest rate
t = time in years

An example of the impact of compound interest on the cost of a nurse call system that cost $120,000 and was financed for 3 years at 12% interest can be shown in Table 2-13.

Interest expense for the nurse call system equals $48,591

Table 2-13 Impact of Compound Interest on Nurse Call System

Period Cost	Beginning Cost (P_0)	$\times$	$(1 + i)$	$=$	Final Cost (V_t)
1	$120,000	$\times$	1.12	$=$	134,400
2	$134,400	$\times$	1.12	$=$	150,528
3	$150,528	$\times$	1.12	$=$	168,591

when the institution pays for it over 3 years at 12% interest compounded annually.

The factor of $(1 + i)^t$ can be called the *compound value interest factor (CVIF)* and can be utilized to calculate the financial impact of compound interest on the purchase of any piece of capital equipment.

CVIF tables are available in most financial texts and can be used as a shortcut in the calculation of the final cost of capital equipment. Table 2-14 is an example of such a CVIF table.

Using a CVIF table, identify the appropriate CVIF factor by finding the appropriate interest rate, or 12%, and trace down the table for the 3-year period. That factor is 1.405. Insert the CVIF of 1.405 into the following equation:

EXAMPLE

$$V_t = P_0(1 + i)^t$$
or
$$V_t = P_0(CVIF)$$

Final cost = beginning cost $\times$ CVIF
Final cost = $120,000 $\times$ 1.405 = $168,600

Table 2-14 shows how interest rates or CVIF tables affect the future value of one of today's dollars at various interest rates.This is an important concept and shows that there is a

Table 2-14 CVIF Table (Compound $1)

Period	8%	9%	10%	12%	14%
1	1.080	1.090	1.100	1.120	1.140
2	1.166	1.186	1.210	1.254	1.300
3	2.260	1.295	1.331	1.405	1.482
4	1.360	1.412	1.464	1.574	1.689
5	1.469	1.539	1.611	1.762	1.925

(Weston JF, Bringham EF: Managerial Finance, 6th ed. Hinsdale, IL, Dryden Press, 1978)

cost involved in borrowing money or paying for something over time or in the future.

This is called the *opportunity cost* of a particular decision, and refers to the fact that there is a real cost associated with making financial decisions at various times and at various interest rates. When certain items are purchased, there is an opportunity cost involved that precludes other financial decisions being made.

PRESENT VALUE

A second concept that flows from compound interest is that of present value or discounting. Determining present value (or discounting, as it is frequently called) is simply the reverse of compounding. The present value of a future cash alternative is calculated by discounting the future commodity by a particular interest rate. The net present value is the worth of the cash flow today.

EXAMPLE OF PRESENT VALUE CALCULATIONS

$$\text{Present value} = \text{final cost} \times \frac{1}{(1 + i)^t}$$

$$P_0 = V_t \frac{1}{(1 + i)^t}$$

$$P_0 = V_t \frac{1}{\text{CVIF}}$$

$$P_0 = \$168,600 \times \frac{1}{1.405} = \frac{\$168,600}{1.0405} = \$120,000$$

$$\frac{1}{\text{CVIF}} = \text{PVIF}_{i,t}$$

These calculations show the reverse of the compounding effect on the original cost of the nurse call system, and shows that $120,000 today, is equal in value to $168,600 in 3 years at a 12% interest rate. Net present value, or discounting, is calculated in a manner opposite to the compound interest method. By altering the original compound interest equation, the net present value equation is developed.

EXAMPLE OF PRESENT VALUE EQUATION

$$\text{Final cost} = \text{present value} \times \text{CVIF}$$
$$V_t = P_0(\text{CVIF})$$

$$\text{Present value} = \text{final cost} \times \frac{1}{\text{CVIF}}$$

$$P_0 = V_t \times \frac{1}{\text{CVIF}}$$

Therefore $P_0 = V_t(\text{PVIF})$

Present value interest factor (PVIF) tables, like the CVIF tables, are available in most financial texts. These tables are used to calculate the present value of future dollars at various interest rates and for various periods of time. Table 2-15 is an example of a PVIF table. The net present value of a financial alternative can be calculated by identifying the PVIF factor in the following manner:

1. Identify the appropriate interest rate.

2. Identify the number of years involved .

3. The PVIF factor is the number at the intersection of the appropriate interest rate and the number of years involved.

4. Solve the net present value equation by inserting the appropriate numbers. $P_0 = V_t(\text{PVIF})$

Discounting allows a decision-maker to put future expenditures in terms of today's dollars, so that intelligent decisions can be made. For example, if a manager were given the following options for paying a medical supply company for supplies received, which method would be preferable?

Alternative 1: Pay $5000 now.

Alternative 2: Make $250 monthly payments for 5 years.

Alternative 3: Make $2000 annual payments for 3 years.

Assuming an interest rate of 9%, which alternative would be the most cost-effective for the head nurse to choose?

Table 2-15   PVIF Tables ($1)

Period	8%	9%	10%	12%	14%
1	.926	.917	.909	.893	.877
2	.857	.842	.826	.797	.769
3	.794	.772	.751	.712	.675
4	.735	.708	.683	.636	.592
5	.681	.650	.621	.567	.519

(Weston JF, Bringham EF: Managerial Finance, 6th ed. Hinsdale, IL, Dryden Press, 1978)

CALCULATIONS

Alternative 1

$P_0 = V_t(PVIF)$
$P_0 = \$5,000$

Alternative 2

$P_0 = V_t(PVIF)$
$P_0 = (\$250 \times 12 \text{ mos.} \times 5 \text{ years}) = \$15,000 \times .650 = \$9,750$
$P_0 = \$9,750$

Alternative 3

$P_0 = V_t(PVIF)$
$P_0 = (\$2,000 \times 3 \text{ years}) = \$6,000 \times .772 = \$4,632$
$P_0 = \$4,632$

When these three options are put into present value terms, it is possible to compare them appropriately and choose the most effective method to pay the medical supply company. Alternative 3 results in the lowest present value payment for the supplies. Therefore, it is the most effective method for paying the bill.

FINANCIAL RATIOS

Ratio analysis is a financial tool that has been commonly used in the business sector to aid management in interpreting financial statements.[8] These ratios are a quantitative way to compare various components of the balance sheet with industry standards. Some of the most frequently used financial ratios include the following:

Current ratio shows the relationship of current assets to current liabilities. It is used as the basic index of liquidity, which identifies the ability of the company to meet its current obligations.

$$\text{Current ratio} = \frac{\text{current assets}}{\text{current liabilities}}$$

Quick ratio/acid test shows the relationship of cash, current receivables, and marketable securities to current liabilities. It indicates a company's ability to discharge its current obligations without the necessity of selling off inventories.

$$\text{Quick ratio} = \frac{\text{cash} + \text{securities} + \text{accounts receivable}}{\text{current liabilities}}$$

Net income to net worth is the percent rate of return received by the owners on their investment.

$$\text{Net income/net worth} = \frac{\text{net income}}{\text{net worth}}$$

Current liabilities to net worth is a percentage indicating the extent to which current creditors are covered by the owners' investment.

$$\text{Current liabilities/net worth} = \frac{\text{current liabilities}}{\text{net worth}}$$

Debt to total assets is the ratio of total long-term debt to total tangible assets. It is used primarily by creditors as an index of protection for their principal.

Net worth to total assets is the ratio of total net worth to total tangible assets, and is used to provide an index of the risk attached to the firm's financial structure. The lower the ratio, the greater the risk is.

$$\frac{\text{Net worth}}{\text{total assets}}$$

Cash to total assets, or the ratio of cash to total tangible assets, is used to provide an index of liquidity and asset allocation balance.

Inventory to total assets is the ratio of inventory holdings to total tangible assets, and is used to provide an index of asset allocation.

Average rate of return is the ratio of the average cash inflow to the average initial investment. It is a measure of the return an investor is receiving on his investment.

Internal rate of return is the discount rate that equates the present value of the expected cash outflows with the present value of the expected inflows. The higher the rate of return, the better the investment is.

SUMMARY

Entire books have been written on the financial management of health care institutions. However, this chapter focused on a few specific key financial concepts and skills that are important for the nurse administrator/manager to understand. The most important concepts are summarized below.

1. The basic financial equation of an organization is *assets = liabilities + owner's equity.*

2. Operating margin is the profit the organization realizes from operations expressed as a percentage. (Operating profits − net patient revenues = operating margin)

3. An institution's cash flow position is greatly influenced by its management of accounts receivable and its credit policies.

4. Owner's equity, net worth, and fund balance are all terms that represent the value or equity the institution owns of the business. (Assets − liabilities = owners' equity, net worth, or fund balance)

5. In cash basis accounting, revenue is recorded when it is actually received. In accrual basis accounting, revenue is recorded when services are delivered, regardless of when the revenue is actually received.

6. Assets are current or liquid when they can be easily and quickly turned into cash.

7. Depreciation is an accounting expense for an organization. It is not a real money expense, but rather an expense on the financial statements that represent the "using up" of capital assets.

8. There are three major deductions that are subtracted from gross patient revenues. The three deductions represent revenue actually lost by the institution and include bad debt, charitable, and contractual allowances.

9. There are essentially two major methods of calculating the value of inventories on the balance sheet: LIFO (last-in, first-out) and FIFO (first-in, first-out).

10. The income statement is a record of the revenue coming into the institution and the expenses leaving the institution.

11. There are essentially two methods of depreciating capital assets: straight-line and accelerated depreciation. Double-declining balance is an example of an accelerated depreciation method.

12. The accounts receivable cycle includes creation of an account receivable, collection, adjustment, and write-off of the account.

13. Capital may be financed through equity or debt. Equity financing includes the issuance of stock and use of retained earnings. Debt financing includes the sale of bonds.

14. The time value concept of money states that a dollar today is worth more than a dollar in the future.

15. The compound interest effect represents the cost of borrowing money to purchase capital assets. The cost of borrowing money increases the final cost of the capital asset.

16. The net present value, or discounted rate, is the reverse of the compounding effect.

17. Financial ratio analysis is a quantitative method of evaluating an organization's financial performance.

18. Current ratio is the basic index of an organization's liquidity, or ability to meet its current obligations.

$$\frac{\text{Current assets}}{\text{current liabilities}}$$

REFERENCES

1. Peters TJ, Waterman R: In Search of Excellence. New York, Harper & Row, 1981
2. JCAH Accreditation Manual, 1985 ed
3. McGee RW: Fundamentals of Accounting and Finance. Englewood, NJ, Prentice-Hall, 1974
4. Lusk E, Lusk J: Financial and Managerial Control: A Health Care Perspective. Rockville, MD, Aspen System, 1979
5. Shillinglaw G, Gordon M, Ronen J: Accounting, A Management Approach, 6th ed. Homewood, IL, Richard D Irwin, 1979
6. Morison LT: "The last word on LIFO--this week! The Journal of Commercial Bank Lending, September 1980
7. Weston JF, Bringham EF: Managerial Finance, 6th ed. Hinsdale, IL, Dryden Press, 1978
8. Almanac of Business and Industrial Ratios, 1979 ed

ADDITIONAL READINGS

1. Holt J, Schaner K: Financing healthcare. Modern Healthcare, June 1982, p 81
2. Staley M, Luciano K: Eight steps to costing nursing services. Nursing Management 15(10):35, 1984

3. How to read a financial report, 4th ed. Merrill, Lynch, Pierce, Fenner, & Smith, Inc.
4. Changing Health Care Policy U.S.A. 1982. Concord, MA, International Health Services, Ltd., 1982
5. Luft HS: National health care expenditures: Where do the dollars go? Inquiry (Blue Cross Association), XII(4):344-363, 1973
6. Sgontz LG: The economics of financing medical care: A review of the literature. Inquiry (Blue Cross Association), IX(4):3-19, Ross 1972
7. Neuman B, Suver J, Zelman W: Financial Management. Owings Mill, MD, National Health Publishing, 1984

3

Introduction to Managerial Cost Accounting and Productivity Principles

COST ACCOUNTING is the financial method of accounting for total costs of a business and then tracking and allocating those costs to the specific product or service produced by the corporation.

The for-profit or private sector has always calculated the cost of producing one unit of service and then used those cost figures to identify their charges or prices. Historically, the health care industry has not identified the total cost of care for a patient for a day, treatment of a particular illness or disease, or performance of a surgical procedure. Within the last decade, however, hospitals have begun to calculate cost per day figures. These figures have not traditionally included all the overhead dollars and normally have not been specific to any particular product line, service, or condition.

In the historical cost-based reimbursement environment, hospitals actually had built-in incentives to inflate their costs because those costs determined reimbursement. Hospitals now must reduce their costs to provide a particular service while maintaining a predetermined level of quality. This calls for the development of a cost-accounting financial system that can calculate actual costs to deliver a particular service. This is accomplished by developing a data base of historical costs and assessing how reductions can be made without reducing the quality of service.

This chapter will outline basic principles and methods for allocating costs and will give specific applications for the nurse manager and executive to use in the health care institution. An overview of principles of productivity and definitions of strategies that the nurse manager can use to increase nursing productivity will then be given.

OBJECTIVES

Upon completing this chapter, the reader will be able to

1. Define basic managerial cost-accounting terminology.
2. Calculate the total cost of providing a particular health care service.
3. Identify various methods for allocating indirect costs to a nursing department.
4. Identify various classifications of hospital costs.
5. Differentiate between transfer and allocation costs.
6. Calculate the total direct departmental cost per unit of service (UOS).
7. Determine the impact of volume on cost per unit of service.
8. Identify the impact of system boundaries on the total cost per UOS.
9. Calculate the break-even point of patients that covers the average operational costs of a unit or hospital.
10. Identify pertinent factors that influence hospital cost per UOS.
11. Identify various strategies to decrease cost per UOS.
12. Define basic productivity terminology and principles to the management of human resources on a nursing unit.

13. Evaluate at least two strategies to increase nursing productivity.

14. Identify at least two different productivity standards for a nursing unit.

15. Develop a productivity standard that includes total direct and indirect nursing costs.

BASIC TERMINOLOGY AND CONCEPTS

A management cost-accounting system ideally consists of two basic components: the historical actual cost-accounting data base and performance standards for each department. The cost-accounting data base provides historical data to identify future cost per unit of service (UOS) goals. Performance standards are developed to measure how a department is managing its resources on an ongoing basis. Performance standards will be addressed toward the end of this chapter. As computers make their way into more acute care institutions, sophisticated cost-accounting systems will become more prevalent.

Specific kinds of costs that need to be identified and understood by the nurse manager are described in the following section.

Fixed costs are costs that are experienced by the hospital regardless of fluctuations in volume or patient days. Fixed costs are the costs that are experienced no matter how many patients are in the hospital. Examples of fixed costs for a nursing unit include the following:

- The salary for the head nurse
- Minimum staffing requirements on the floor
- The cost of the infection control nurse, quality assurance nurse, director of nursing, and so on

Examples of fixed costs for the entire hospital include the following:

- The expense of the medical records department
- The cost of administration
- The cost of the human resource department
- The cost of depreciation
- The cost of insurance
- The cost of financing capital projects

Figure 3-1 shows how fixed costs are represented on a graph that includes cost and/or revenue on one axis and volume or patient days on the other axis.

Variable costs are costs that are a function of volume or patient days. Variable costs are over and above the fixed costs. Examples of variable costs for a nursing unit include the following:

- Nurse staffing by acuity above minimum staffing pattern
- Medical supplies for specific patients
- Linen costs
- Food costs

Figure 3-2 shows how variable costs are represented graphically over fixed costs and how they vary with volume. Fixed costs plus variable costs equal total costs.

Total costs are the sum of fixed and variable costs, as shown in Figure 3-2.

Cost per unit of service or *unit cost* is the cost to produce a single product or unit of service. The unit of service for inpatient care is the *patient day*. Examples of units of service for specific departments in a hospital and other health care systems are shown in Table 3-1.

There are two basic cost-accounting methods: direct costing and full costing.

Direct costing is a method of accounting for all costs

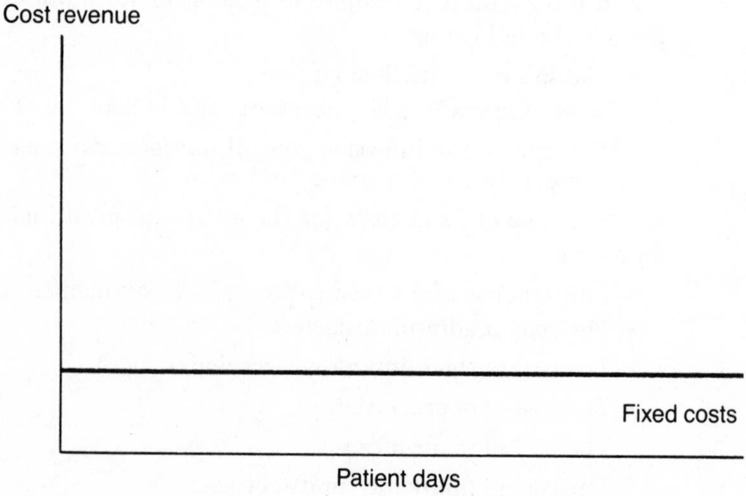

Cost revenue

Fixed costs

Patient days

Figure 3-1. *Fixed costs.*

Costs, revenue

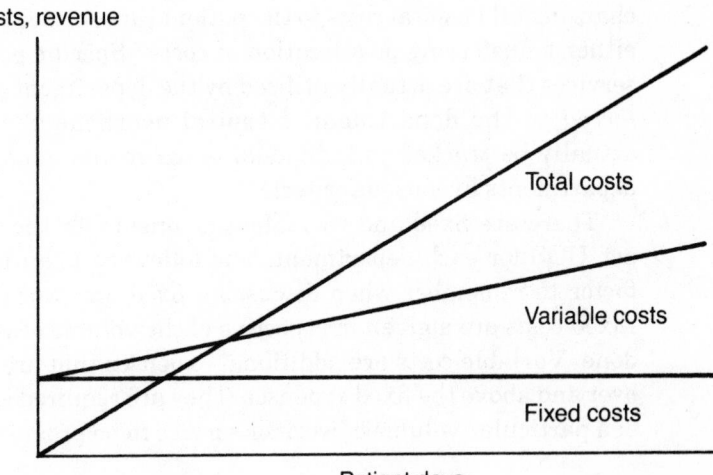

Patient days

Figure 3-2. *Total costs.*

incurred directly by a specific cost center or department. Direct cost accounting compares a department's actual outflows or direct costs with its inflows or revenue from patient care services delivered on that particular unit.

Full costing is the cost-accounting method that includes the direct departmental costs, as well as the indirect costs, that are transferred and/or allocated to the department. The strength of the full-costing method is that it takes total hospital costs into account. Its weakness lies in the fact that some of the indirect costs allocated to a specific department may be irrelevant to the actual revenue produced by the patient care service provided by that department.

Full costing is determining the total cost of providing patient care services for the hospital, and is the process of

Table 3-1   Examples of Units of Service for Health Care

Department	Unit of Service
Radiology	Procedures
Home health agency	Home visits
Surgery department	Surgery minutes
	Anesthesia minutes
Recovery room	Outpatient recoveries
	Inpatient recoveries
Maintenance department	Work orders
Dietary department	Meals

charging all hospital costs to the patient care service centers by either transferring or allocation of costs.[1] Specific products or services that are actually utilized by the department are *transferred* to the department. Hospital overhead that cannot actually be tracked to individual departments is *allocated* to departments by various criteria.

There are fixed and variable components for the total cost per UOS for each department. The following is an important factor to remember when discussing fixed and variable costs: Fixed costs are a given irrespective of the volume of work to be done. Variable costs are additional expenses that are required over and above the fixed expenses. They are required as a result of a particular volume of work or service to be provided.

DIRECT AND INDIRECT COSTS

Another concept in cost accounting is that of direct and indirect cost relationships. In a hospital, *direct costs* are costs that are directly connected with the delivery of patient care services. The cost of nursing salaries and the cost of medical supplies for patients are direct costs.[2]

Indirect costs are necessary but not directly related to the delivery of specific patient care services. Examples of indirect costs include the following:

- Director of nursing's salary
- Engineering department expenses
- Billing department expenses
- Medical records department
- Cost of administration

These indirect costs are for support services that are required for the total functioning of the hospital.

Indirect costs are attached to fixed costs by transfer or allocation. An indirect cost may be transferred to a department based on the department's actual utilization of the service or product. For example, linen costs are transferred to a specific nursing unit based on the actual amount of linen the unit uses for patients.

Allocation of indirect costs is not based on actual utilization but rather assigned to a particular department based on a specific criterion. An example of the allocation of indirect costs is the allocation of employee benefits to departmental budgets based on the number of full-time equivalents (FTEs) in each department (*e.g.*, workmen's compensation and health care benefits are allocated to a particular department based on the number of their approved FTEs).

SAMPLE CALCULATIONS

Total hospital cost of benefits ÷ total hospital FTEs = cost per FTE
Cost/FTE × departmental FTEs = departmental allocation
for benefits

$900,000 ÷ 500 FTEs = $1,800/FTE
$1,800 × 32 FTEs (ICU) = $57,600 (allocation for ICU)

Transfer and Allocation of Indirect Costs

Different indirect costs are allocated to different departments or cost centers based on various criteria that are determined by hospital administration.[3] Examples of criteria for allocating indirect expenses to patient care areas are shown in Table 3-2.

A major reason for developing a cost-accounting system in a hospital is to maintain management control over expenses. It is important to note that direct costs and transferable costs are fairly controllable by the manager, whereas allocated indirect costs are not really under the control of the manager. It is crucial for managers to understand the costs involved for the entire organization in providing patient care services. By allocating as many indirect costs as possible to individual departmental budgets, the manager achieves a more complete and comprehensive understanding of the institution's total expenses. By only including the direct costs for a department in the budget, the manager and staff have a very limited perspective and concept of the costs involved in the delivery of patient care services.

Indirect costs are transferred or allocated to specific departments for two major reasons. The transfer or allocation of costs allows all managers to participate and be responsible for the control of overhead expenses. For example, by transferring maintenance costs to repair holes in the walls, beds, blood pressure machines, patient furniture, and so on, the nursing man-

---

Table 3-2   Transfer and/or Allocation Criteria for Indirect Costs

Department	Criteria
Medical records	1. Percentage of time spent processing charts for each floor.
	2. Divide total costs by patient charts processed per year to determine cost per patient record. Allocate cost to units by number of patients cared for on each unit.
Maintenance	1. Cost of work orders times the number of work orders per unit.
	2. Square feet of department as a percentage of the entire hospital.
	3. Routine cost for maintenance of a department plus the actual cost for special projects.
Employee health and benefits	1. Divide total hospital costs for benefits by total number of FTEs. Allocate to units by the number of departmental FTEs.
	2. Allocate based on gross department salary dollars.
Housekeeping	1. By hours of service in a department.
	2. By square feet in a department for routine cleaning and then charge for specific services.
	3. By frequency and nature of cleaning services.
Administration	1. By FTEs in a department.
	2. By gross departmental expenses.
	3. By hours of support to each department.
	4. Divide administrators' salaries by the number of departments supervised.
Human resource department	1. By FTEs in department.
	2. By hours of service delivered to each department.

---

ager and staff become very aware of the cost of repairing these items. Unit staff and management take responsibility for maintaining their environment when they are fiscally accountable via their unit budgets. The manager and staff become accountable for the maintenance of their unit because the cost to maintain it is actually reflected in their budget and monthly variance report. There is an incentive to take this responsibility seriously because the nursing manager is evaluated on his or her fiscal management of the unit.

A second reason for transferring and allocating the cost of overhead is to give the manager a truer picture of the total costs required in providing patient care services. When a department manager has access to the figures for overhead costs and can see what the institution pays for expenses such as administration, depreciation, finance costs, data processing services, legal fees, utilities, maintenance of medical records, and public relations, he or she has a better understanding of the magnitude of the expenses that are required to operate a hospital.

When a hospital does not transfer or allocate indirect costs to departmental budgets, it is easy for department directors to have a skewed picture of their revenue and expense status. For example, department managers prepare monthly variance reports comparing actual volume, revenue, and expenses with their budgeted figures. If their expense figures do not include any transferred or allocated indirect costs, the department's profits or contribution margin figures appear overstated and more significant than is actually the case. Table 3-3 shows an example of a medical-surgical nursing unit's variance report for a specific month without any transferred or allocated costs. The second example (Table 3-4) shows the same unit for the same month with some transfer costs included.

By including the transferred indirect costs for dietary, maintenance, linen, and housekeeping services, the unit's contribution dropped from 71% to 67%. If overhead costs for administration, medical records, financing costs, depreciation, and so on were allocated to the unit, the profit contribution would decrease even further.

Table 3-3 Contribution Margin of Medical–Surgical Unit Without Transfer Costs

	Month
Units of service	753
Revenue	$225,208
Expenses	
Salaries	61,390
Medical supplies	1,835
Nonmedical supplies	1,067
Purchased services	
Maintenance	
Equipment rentals	
Dues and travel	185
Interdepartmental transfers	
Other	
Total expenses	$ 64,477
Unit contribution	$160,731
Contribution margin	71%

Table 3-4   Contribution Margin of Medical–Surgical Unit With Transfer Costs

	Month
Units of service	753
Revenue	$225,208
Expenses	
Salaries	61,390
Medical supplies	1,835
Nonmedical supplies	1,067
Purchased services	
Maintenance	3,008
Equipment rentals	
Dues and travel	185
Interdepartmental transfers	5,320
Physician compensation	
Other	
Total expenses	$ 72,805
Unit contribution	$152,403
Contribution margin	67%

DEFINING THE BOUNDARIES OF THE COST-ACCOUNTING SYSTEM

It is important to define the boundaries included in a managerial cost-accounting system because the boundaries determine the detail of the costs identified. Many hospitals have effectively defined the cost per UOS on a departmental basis or the average cost of a patient day. They have identified average patient day cost by dividing the total hospital budget by the number of patient days actually experienced.

SAMPLE CALCULATIONS

Total hospital expenses ÷ patient days = average cost/patient day
$20 million   ÷   25,000   = $800/patient day

Table 3-5 shows how a medical surgical nursing department calculates average direct costs per UOS.

Some hospitals allocate the indirect costs of linen, dietary, and maintenance services to each individual unit. Table 3-6 shows how the cost per UOS is affected if the same medical-surgical unit would have those particular costs transferred to it for the same month.

When the indirect costs for linen, dietary, and maintenance services are transferred to the patient care unit, the cost per

Table 3-5 Direct Cost per Unit of Service

	Month
Units of service	753
Expenses	
Salaries	$61,390
Medical supplies	1,835
Nonmedical supplies	1,067
Purchased services	
Maintenance	
Equipment rentals	
Dues and travel	185
Interdepartmental transfers	
Physician compensation	
Other	
Total expenses	$64,477
Expense/Unit of service	$85.62

UOS increases from $85.62 to $96.68. This cost per UOS does not include the indirect overhead of administration, medical records department services, depreciation, financing costs, and so on. When those overhead costs are allocated to the department, cost per UOS will increase even more.

The cost per UOS varies depending on whether management is considering only the costs directly experienced by the department or whether expenses include services provided to the department, such as linen, maintenance, and other services. The boundaries of the system included in the cost-account-

Table 3-6 Cost per Unit of Service with Transferred Costs

	Month
Units of service	753
Expenses	
Salaries	$61,390
Medical supplies	1,835
Nonmedical supplies	1,067
Purchased services	
Maintenance	3,008
Equipment rentals	
Dues and travel	185
Interdepartmental transfers	5,320
Physician compensation	
Other	
Total expenses	$72,805
Cost per UOS	$96.68

ing data system determines what the cost accounting data are actually measuring.

Before comparing costs for patient care services of hospitals and/or departments, it is important to understand the costs actually included in the data. This can be determined by answering the following questions:

- Does the system include only the direct costs of the department?
- Does the system include some or all of the transfer costs for supplies and/or services utilized by the department?
- Does the system include the allocation of costs for all hospital overhead?

As hospital accounting systems become more sophisticated and automated, they can expand the boundaries and scope of the data included in their cost-accounting management systems. Hospitals usually progress in their management cost-accounting system capability in the following manner:

1. Cost per UOS is calculated by departments based on their direct costs.

2. Costs for linen, maintenance, and dietary services, as well as employee benefits, are transferred or allocated to individual departments.

3. Costs for advertising, education, and biomedical services are transferred to individual departments.

4. Costs for administration, medical records services, depreciation, and so on are allocated to departments.

5. Product line managers are accountable for quality, cost, marketing, and so on for individual products and services.

BREAK-EVEN ANALYSIS

Break-even analysis is an analysis of the cost, volume, and profit of a particular product or service used to assist managers in their decision making.[4] The *break-even point* is the volume of a product or service that equals predetermined cost or profit goals. The volume of patient days that equal the break-even point is the number of patients in the hospital on a given day that are required to cover the cost of the average daily operations of the hospital. Break-even analysis can be used by the nurse manager or nurse executive for the following situations in the hospital:

1. To identify the number of procedures that would need to be done to pay for a piece of capital equipment

---

SAMPLE CALCULATIONS

Cost of laser for surgery = $750,000
Average charge for use of laser (no other costs included) = $950
Break-even point or number of procedures needed to be done to pay for laser = 789 procedures

A hospital would pay for the laser after doing 789 cases. The hospital would begin making a profit from the piece of equipment after doing the 789 cases (not including other revenue realized from the patients' hospitalizations).

---

2. To identify the minimum number of patients on a nursing unit that will cover the direct unit costs of minimum staffing requirements

---

SAMPLE CALCULATIONS

Minimum Staffing on Nursing Unit

Shift	Number of Nurses	Hours
7–3	2	16
3–11	2	16
11–7	2	16
	Head nurse (40 hours ÷ 7 days)	5.7
	Total =	53.7

Minimum hrs ÷ productivity standard = break-even point
53.7 hrs ÷ 5 HPPD = 10.7 patients (break-even)

OR

Total cost for minimum staffing ÷ budgeted cost/UOS = break-even point
53.7 hr × $12/hr ÷ 5 HPPD × $12/hr = 10.7 patients
$644.40 ÷ $60 = 10.7 patients

The nursing unit must maintain at least 10.7 patients on the unit at all times to pay for the direct costs of the minimum staffing for the unit. If the patient census drops below this point (10.7 patients), the unit will experience higher costs than the productivity standard of 5 HPPD. If such conditions should occur for a period of time, the hospital would experience greater expenses than planned for in the budget and the profit margin would decrease.

Figure 3-3 shows the break-even point or number of patients per unit based on the minimum staffing requirements.

Break-even analysis or cost-volume-profit analysis includes

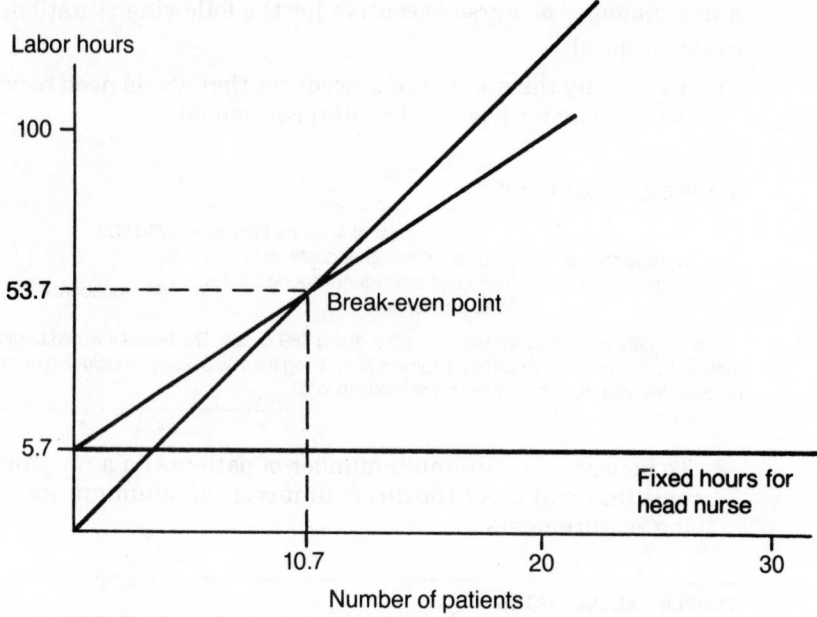

Figure 3-3.   *Break-even calculations for minimum staffing.*

the following assumptions that the nurse manager should understand:

1. Costs can be broken down into fixed and variable costs.
2. Fixed costs remain essentially constant despite changes in volume or patient census.
3. Variable costs fluctuate with volume or patient census.
4. Charges for patient care services are considered a constant over the period of time being considered.
5. The cost of expense factors such as salaries is held constant over the predetermined time period.
6. Efficiency and productivity standards are held constant over the time in question.
7. Revenue and expense behavior can be considered linear with changes in volume.

Margin of safety is the excess of budgeted or actual revenue over the break-even patient revenue figures.[1]

A hospital's margin of safety is the number of patients or amount of patient revenue that is in excess of the break-even figures.

SAMPLE CALCULATIONS

Break-even point + margin of safety = budgeted patient census
83 patients   +   19 patients   =   102 budgeted census

A 150-bed hospital has calculated that its break-even point is a daily census of 86 patients. This means that when 83 patients are in the hospital, the average revenue from those 83 patients equals or covers the average daily expenses required to run the entire hospital.

Annual operating expenses = $30,000,000
Average daily patient revenue = $995
Average daily operating expenses ($30,000,000 for 365 days) = $82,192

Average daily operating expense ÷ average revenue/patient = break-even census
$82,192   ÷ $995   =   83 patients

As long as the census stays above 83 patients and expenses do not increase, the hospital will not suffer a loss. If, however, the census falls below 83 patients, the hospital will need to reduce its daily operating expenses or suffer a loss.

A declining inpatient census is one of the most significant problems CEOs are facing in the 1980s.[3] Therefore, it is very important for all of the hospital's managers to understand the concept and implications of the break-even analysis.

In the following example, every patient above the break-even point of 83 patients results in potential profit for the hospital. By budgeting for a daily average census of 102, the hospital is budgeting for an average daily profit of $18,905, or an annual profit ("bottom line") of $6,900,325.

SAMPLE CALCULATIONS

Average revenue/patient day × safety margin = gross profit
$995   ×   19 patients   = $18,905
$995 × 19 patients   ×   365 days   = $6,900,325

If an institution is having census problems, it is important that fixed costs be as low as possible. By reducing fixed costs it is possible actually to reduce the break-even point. When census is a problem, it is helpful for management to move as many fixed costs into variable costs as possible to reduce the break-even point.

The next case example will show how a nursing executive can reduce the break-even point for patient census and occupancy on a nursing unit.

SAMPLE CALCULATIONS

A medical–surgical nursing unit has the following fixed costs as a result of fixed staffing and nursing administration overhead. The unit has a productivity standard of 6 HPPD for total nursing care and has 26 beds.

Roles	Hours Per Day
Head nurse (40 hr ÷ 7 days)	5.7
7–3 Shift	
2 Licensed nurses	16
1 Ward secretary	8
1 Nurse aide	8
3–11 Shift	
2 Licensed nurses	16
1 Ward secretary	8
1 Nurse aide	8
11–7 Shift	
2 Licensed nurses	16
1 Nurse aide	8
Nursing administration overhead	10
Total	103.7

103.7 hr ÷ 6 HPPD standard = 17.3 patients to break-even

Nursing Administration Overhead Calculations	Hours Per Week
VP nursing	40
Assistant DON	40
VP's secretary	40
Staffing secretaries (16 hr × 7 days)	112
2 Clinical specialists	80
Infection control nurse	40
Quality assurance nurse	40
House supervision (24 hr × 7 days)	168
Total weekly nursing overhead	560

560 hr ÷ 7 days ÷ 8 units = 10 hr overhead/day/nursing unit

This nursing unit needs to maintain 17.3 patients in the unit at all times to cover the fixed expense of minimum staffing and nursing administration overhead. Since it is a 26-bed unit, it will break-even from the perspective of nursing direct and indirect salary costs at 66% occupancy.

As inpatient census in medical-surgical units declines, it is important for the nurse executive to be able to decrease the fixed salary costs of direct and indirect nursing care. This can be accomplished either by decreasing fixed overhead positions or moving fixed salary costs into variable costs and adding staff when census increases.

Most hospitals do not include the indirect costs of nursing administration in their patient care productivity standards, over and above the unit manager or head nurse role. However, by not including that overhead in the actual patient care standard, managers get a false sense of the "true" costs of nursing in their hospital. The overhead costs of nursing "support" roles identified in the previous case example are essentially not under the control of the unit manager or head nurse. However, by integrating the nursing administration overhead costs into the individual nursing unit budgets, the nurse executive can get a better sense of the true total costs of providing nursing care in the institution. When budget reductions need to be made for organizational survival, it is important that the nurse executive look at the cost and benefits of the overhead of the nursing administration support roles, as well as the patient care providers.

The impact of moving fixed costs into variable costs to reduce the break-even point in times of reduced census will be discussed next. If some of the nursing administration overhead roles and the minimum staffing patterns are reduced on the same unit, it is possible to see the impact on the number of patients that need to be maintained on the unit to break-even.

SAMPLE CALCULATIONS

Role	Hours Per Day
Changes in Minimum Staffing and Nursing Administration	
Head Nurse	5.7
7–3 Shift: licensed nurses	16.0
3–11 Shift: 2 licensed nurses	16.0
11–7 Shift: 2 licensed nurses	16.0
Nursing administration overhead	5.1
Total hours	61.8

61.8 hr ÷ 6 HPPD standard = 10.3 patients to break-even

Changes in Nursing Administration Overhead	Hours Per Week
VP nursing	40
ADON	40
Nursing secretary	40
Staffing secretary	40
Off-shift supervision (16 hr × 7 days)	128
Total hours	288

288 hr ÷ 7 days ÷ 8 units = 5.1 hr nursing overhead per day

The second part of this example shows how the nurse executive reduced the minimum patients the unit needs to maintain from 17.3 to 10.3 patients. As patient census increases over 10.3, the nurse manager can add additional variable care givers and/or a ward secretary to manage the workload. A good cost reduction plan takes into consideration the nursing administration overhead, as well as the staffing patterns on the individual units to maintain quality while reducing expenses. This nurse executive reduced nursing administration overhead by 50% by reassigning specific nursing responsibilities and tasks.

In this particular case, the nurse executive reduced the nursing administration overhead by implementing the following changes:

1. The nine head nurses who report to the VP each takes a turn functioning as the day supervisor on Saturday and Sunday. Because there are nine of them, each functions in this role only once every 2 months.

2. The staffing secretary function was assumed by the unit assistant head nurses and the off-shift supervisors on the 3-11 and 11-7 shifts. This reduced the hours for staffing secretary coverage from 112 hours per week to 40 hours per week. The staffing secretary function was maintained during the day shift Monday through Friday.

3. The two clinical nurse specialist roles were eliminated by attrition, and the head nurses and assistant head nurses were given the responsibility for clinical supervision of direct care on each unit.

   In many hospitals, the number and amount of positions in nursing administration make it fairly easy to make reductions without adversely affecting the quality of care. The traditional nursing hierarchy of the 1960s and 1970s is a very expensive organizational model, and one that hospitals cannot afford to maintain in the 1980s and 1990s. The nurse executive needs to identify functions, needs, and responsibilities for various nursing positions for the purpose of potentially combining, deleting, and/or shifting selected nursing functions.

4. The quality assurance function was assumed by the individual nursing units, and staff nurses began auditing nursing care standards on a monthly basis. The head nurses submitted those studies to the quality assurance committee on an ongoing basis.

5. The infection control function was assumed by the assistant director of nursing. The organizational structure before and after is represented in Figures 3-4 and 3-5.

METHODS OF DECREASING COST PER UOS

As prospective contracting and competition between hospitals increase, pressure to decrease costs will continue. An effective method for a nurse executive to stay on top of nursing costs

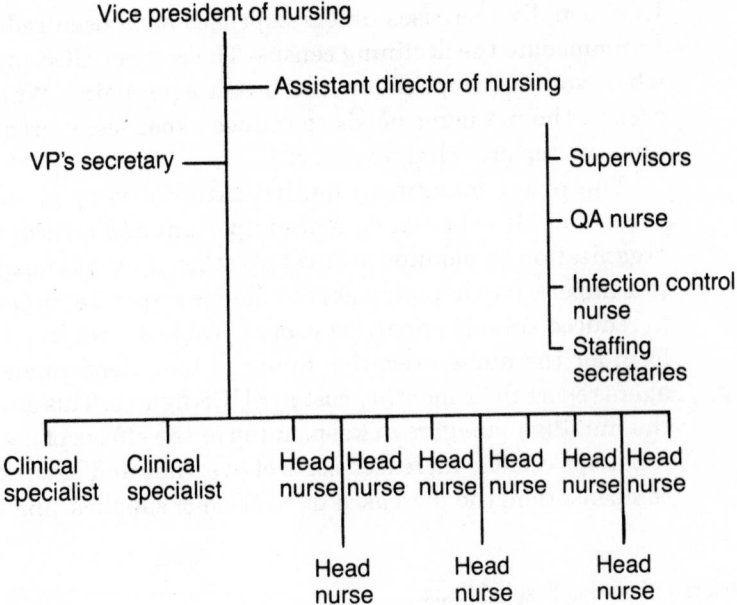

Figure 3-4. *Nursing management structure before reductions.*

includes the continuous monitoring of cost per UOS. Cost per UOS becomes very important because patient census is becoming more unpredictable and crucial. As revenue per patient day drops, it is important for the administrative nurse to understand the cost of delivering nursing care by patient day or UOS. As volume of service or patient census declines, the cost per

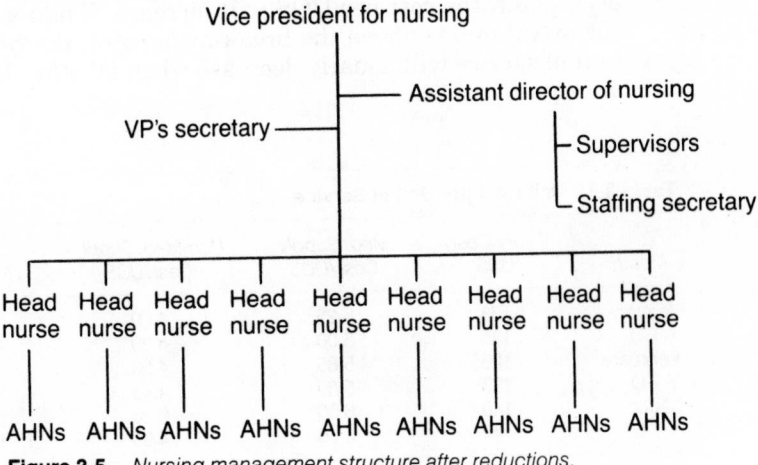

Figure 3-5. *Nursing management structure after reductions.*

UOS usually increases unless expenses have been reduced to accommodate the declining census. The cost per UOS increases when volume drops below the break-even point. When this occurs, the manager needs to reduce expenses, increase volume, or stop providing the service.

The profit margin in health care delivery is steadily decreasing. It is becoming more important and critical for the organization to monitor unit costs rather than total expenses. It is imperative that managers be able to respond appropriately to reduced volume or patient census. Table 3-7 shows a sample form for the nurse executive to use to have department managers report their monthly cost per UOS figures. This allows all the nursing managers to keep on top of the effects of declining inpatient census, increased costs of overtime and of workmen's compensation, the increased utilization of supplies, and so on.

Factors Influencing Hospital Costs

There are various factors influencing health care costs and departmental cost per UOS figures that should be identified and understood by nurse managers and administrators. These factors include the following:

- Patient census, occupancy, or volume of service produced. When referring to patient census, it is important for the total fixed and indirect expenses of the hospital to be covered by the revenue that is experienced from the average patient census. If patient census is lower than the break-even point, the cost per UOS will increase. If patient census or volume is above the break-even point, the cost per unit of service will usually decrease when all other factors are equal.

Table 3-7   Unit Cost per Unit of Service

Month	Salary Cost/ UOS	Med. Supply Cost/UOS	Non-Med. Supply Cost/UOS	Total Cost/UOS
January	133	5.25	4.00	142.25
Y-T-D	135	5.00	4.20	144.20
February	123	5.85	4.50	133.35
Y-T-D	133	5.50	4.45	142.95
March	140	6.00	6.25	152.25
Y-T-D	144	5.70	4.85	154.55

- Physician practice patterns affect the cost per UOS. When physicians overutilize critical care and telemetry units, the high salary costs of these labor-intensive units increase the average cost per patient day for the hospital. When physicians order many laboratory tests, treatments, medications, and so on, the average cost per patient day increases. In the current prospective reimbursement environment of DRGs, the length of stay is very important in determining the cost per case of a particular admission. When cost per case increases as a result of length of stay, the profit margin of the hospital may be significantly reduced.

- Productivity affects departmental cost per UOS, as well as hospital-wide average cost per patient day. This is due to the labor-intensive nature of patient care services. When labor or salaries exceed predetermined standards, costs are significantly affected because of the high salary costs of professional nurses, pharmacists, dieticians, social workers, and others. Salaries account for approximately 50% to 60% of total hospital costs. Increases in salaries significantly impact cost per UOS figures. (Productivity will be discussed in greater detail later in this chapter.)

- Overutilization of supplies and lost charges impact departmental cost per UOS. In the current health care environment, it is important for nurses and nurse managers to monitor and utilize supplies wisely and prudently.

- Contract rates for hospital supplies impact the cost per patient day. Group purchasing agreements through organizations and associations such as American Hospital Association, Volunteer Hospitals of America, and others significantly decrease the cost of supplies such as radiology film, pharmaceuticals, paper products, sutures, medical supplies, and food. By purchasing these items at lower, group-purchasing prices, the average cost per patient day can be reduced or at least maintained.

- Employee health and benefit utilization affects hospital costs significantly. Excessive utilization of health benefits and/or benefits such as workmen's compensation increase hospital costs because of the complete overhead nature of the expense. Anything that an institution can do to decrease these outlays is well worth the effort to decrease hospital costs.

Other factors influencing hospital costs include the following:

- Percentage of MediCaid and Medicare patients

- The hospital's credit rating, which determines financing costs
- Size and age of the hospital, which determines the overhead costs for maintenance, utilities, and housekeeping
- The amount of medical research an institution is involved in
- The specific programs and services at a hospital, which can determine its costs per patient day. For example, if a hospital operates a heart transplant program, it will have significantly higher costs than a hospital that provides routine medical and surgical care.

DEVELOPMENT OF MANAGERIAL COST-ACCOUNTING SYSTEMS IN HOSPITALS

Trumond Esmond, President of a health care financial consulting firm in Barrington, Illinois, stresses the need for hospitals to assemble total costs for a comprehensive financial system.[4] Some hospitals are turning to standard cost accounting systems, while others are adapting to an existing system borrowed from the manufacturing industry.

One of the questions facing hospital administrators concerns the level of sophistication or complexity to obtain in a cost-accounting system. The answer to this question depends on the size of the institution, resources available, and leadership insight. Regardless of the level of sophistication, the system must be able to break down costs to the procedure level or unit of service level for each department.

A second key component of a cost-accounting system is the development of engineered productivity standards for all hospital departments. William Nelson, Senior Vice-President of Finance for Intermountain Health Care, Inc. (IHC), Salt Lake City, estimates that 95% of all hospitals lack productivity standards. Intermountain Health Care, Inc. may have one of the most advanced cost-accounting systems for hospitals in the country. This multi-hospital system has developed standard costs for each procedure at each individual hospital in the system.[4]

Standard cost accounting is the managerial cost-accounting method that identifies the total or standard cost for each hospital procedure. The standard cost for a procedure such as a laboratory test or an obstetrical delivery includes the following component costs:

- Variable overhead
- Fixed overhead
- Allocation of depreciation
- Fixed labor costs
- Variable labor costs
- Variable supply costs

Standard costing allows the hospital to identify procedural standard costs and thus make intelligent decisions about contracting, discount pricing, expansion or reduction of a specific service, and productivity for an individual department.[5]

Two examples of the breakdown of the standard costing for a particular procedure are displayed in Figure 3-6 and Table 3-8.

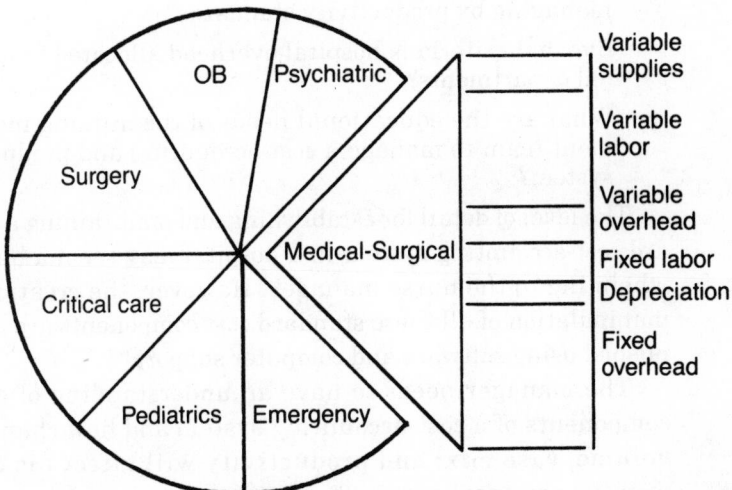

Figure 3-6. *Break-down of standard costs.*
Fixed overhead = allocation of administration, medical records, data processing, insurance
Fixed labor costs = head nurse's salary, minimum staffing, allocation for nursing administration overhead
Variable overhead = cost of utilities, maintenance, employee benefits
Variable labor costs = cost of acuity-determined staffing, overtime, call-in pay, sick-time pay, etc.
Variable supplies = cost of admit kits, medical supplies, nonmedical supplies, food, linen

Table 3-8   Standard Cost Break-Down of an Emergency Room Visit

	Labor Cost	Supply Cost	Other Cost	Depreciation	Dept. Total	Hospital Overhead	Total Cost
Fixed cost	10.10	1.52	1.21	4.20	17.03	9.83	26.86
Variable cost	14.20	4.53			18.73	3.18	21.91
Total cost	25.30	6.05	1.21	4.20	36.76	13.01	49.77

The nurse executive needs to become familiar with the cost-accounting system used in the institution by seeking answers to the following questions:

- How are direct costs, transfer costs, and allocated indirect costs defined and integrated into the individual departmental budgets?
- What level of detail is required?
- Are the productivity standards for nursing procedures valid? How were they developed?
- Is nursing management prepared for and committed to managing by productivity standards?
- By what criteria is hospital overhead allocated to individual departments?
- What are the educational needs of the nursing management team to manage a cost-accounting and productivity system?

The level of detail for establishing and maintaining a standard cost-accounting system in a hospital may seem a bit overwhelming to the nurse manager. However, the creation and manipulation of all these standard cost components are accomplished using software and computer support.

The manager needs to have an understanding of all the components of a cost-accounting system and how changes in volume, case mix, and productivity will affect his or her monthly variance reports. The nurse manager is expected to be able to identify strategies to increase productivity and/or decrease fixed or variable costs to maintain the organization's viability.

Staley and Luciano identified eight steps in the actual costing of nursing services.[6] They effectively identified a methodology for determining the direct costs of providing nursing care to patients on a particular unit. They stopped short, however, of the level of detail required in the current health care environment. A critique of their article includes the following points:

1. They do not discuss what is included in the indirect expenses or overhead items allocated to the individual departments. The current health care environment demands that all indirect costs be allocated to the departments and be attached to revenue-producing procedures or services.

2. Staley and Luciano calculate salary expense per hour for a patient's entire length of stay at the same rate. This level of detail is not adequate. Salary cost per hour should be calculated by unit. For example, the salary cost for nursing care in the ICU is more expensive per hour than that on a medical-surgical unit because of the staffing mix.

3. The article does not seem to deal with the cost of nursing administration as an indirect overhead cost of patient care. Traditionally, nursing administration has been a large overhead cost center that really needs to be considered and calculated as a component of the standard cost of a patient day.

INTRODUCTION TO PRODUCTIVITY

Productivity measures how efficiently labor resources are utilized in producing a good or service. In nursing, productivity is defined as a measure of the efficiency of human resources utilized in the delivery of patient care services. John Kendrick defines productivity as the "relationship between output (O) of goods and services and the inputs (I) of resources, human and nonhuman, used in the production process."[7] This relationship can be expressed as

$$\frac{\text{Output}}{\text{Input}} = \text{Productivity}$$

The higher the numerical value of this relationship, the greater is the productivity or efficiency. Individual managers and organizations need to be concerned about the productivity of their departments and/or organization because of the following factors:

- Productivity is a key strategy to strengthen the competitive position of the hospital.
- High productivity conserves valuable resources.
- Productivity helps counteract the effects of inflation.
- Improvements in productivity help an organization deal with growth and increased demand for services.

Productivity is measured against a productivity standard. A *productivity standard* is a quantifiable period of time needed to accomplish a specific procedure or task. The productivity measures that are most utilized in hospitals are called *labor productivity standards*. A labor productivity standard is the output per work hour, or a measure of the

$$\frac{\text{Output in work hours}}{\text{Input of labor hours}}$$

In a nursing department, the output in work hours is determined by multiplying the number of patient days or units of service produced times the established standard for the unit.

SAMPLE CALCULATIONS

Patient days   × unit standard =   output in work hours
280 Patient days ×   5 HPPD   = 1,400 work hours (output)

Productivity is calculated by dividing the work output by the actual hours worked or labor input.

SAMPLE CALCULATIONS

$$\frac{\text{Output of work hours}}{\text{input of worked hours}} = \text{productivity}$$

$$\frac{1,400 \text{ hours required}}{1,325 \text{ hours worked}} = 105\% \text{ productivity}$$

In this example, the nursing staff was 104% productive. That is, they cared for the patients with 5% less staff than the acuity/classification system or standard required.

In their recent articles in *Hospitals,* Harju and Sabatino relate that productivity improvements in nursing, laboratory services, surgery, medical records, and radiology are "very important" for a hospital to thrive in the prospective reimbursement environment.[3]

For a long time, nursing has had productivity measures in the form of acuity systems or patient classification systems. A *patient classification system* is a method of classifying patients into a group or category based on some specific criteria. An *acu-*

ity system is a method of classifying patients by severity of illness to provide appropriate nurse staffing, level, and professional mix.[8]

All hospital departments should have productivity standards. Productivity standards are important to ensure that all hospital departments are operating as efficiently and productively as possible.

Productivity standards are usually developed using industrial engineering methods that utilize observation of operations and time and motion studies. After these studies are completed, the data are manipulated to determine an appropriate standard for a unit.

Nursing Productivity Standards

In the nursing department, hours per patient day (HPPD) is the criterion most commonly used as a productivity standard. Patient classification systems assign various HPPD figures to each acuity level or patient classification. Then organizations measure nursing productivity in one of two ways:

1. Nursing productivity is measured by comparing actual staffing hours with staffing hours required by the patient classification system. In this method, there is no average HPPD standard that needs to be maintained. Nurse staffing needs to approximate staffing hours required by the classification system.

EXAMPLE

A critical care unit has two patient acuity levels. Acuity 1 calls for 24 HPPD, and the patient requires 1 : 1 nursing care. Acuity 2 calls for 12 HPPD, and the patient receives 1 : 2 nurse to patient staffing. The standard for this unit also includes 29.7 fixed hours per day (HPD) to account for 24 hours of monitor technician coverage and 5.7 hours for head nurse coverage (40 hours ÷ 7 days = 5.7 hours per day). The productivity standard for this critical care unit is written like this:

Critical Care Standard

Number of acuity 1 patients = _____ × 24 HPPD = _____ hours required
Number of acuity 2 patients = _____ × 12 HPPD = _____ hours required
Fixed HPD for indirect nursing care = 29.7 hours
Total required HPPD = _____

Sample Calculations

On a specific day, the unit has three acuity 1 patients and eight acuity 2 patients. The unit was staffed with the following personnel:

Shift	Staff	Hours
7–3	7 Nurses	56.0
	1 Head nurse	5.7

	1 Monitor technician	8.0
3–11	7 Nurses	56.0
	1 Monitor technician	8.0
11–7	6 Nurses	48.0
	1 Monitor technician	8.0
Total hours worked		189.7

The unit's productivity is calculated in the following manner:

$$\text{Number of acuity1} = 3 \times 24 \text{ HPPD} = \quad 72.0 \text{ hours}$$
$$\text{Number of acuity 2} = 8 \times 12 \text{ HPPD} = \quad 96.0 \text{ hours}$$
$$\text{Fixed HPD for indirect care} \qquad = \underline{\quad 29.7} \text{ hours}$$
$$\text{Total required HPPD} \qquad = 197.7 \text{ hours}$$

$$\text{Productivity} = \frac{\text{hours required}}{\text{hours worked}} = \frac{197.7}{189.7} = 104\%$$

A productivity of 104% means the nursing staff was 4% more productive than called for by the standard. The nursing staff cared for patients with 4% fewer resources than called for by the standard. A productivity below 100% means that the unit used more nursing resources to care for a particular group of patients than the standard required. A productivity above 100% means that the unit utilized less labor resources than the standard required to care for the patients.

2. The second example of a nursing standard is exhibited by an average HPPD standard for patient care and a fixed number of hours for indirect labor cost for a particular unit.

EXAMPLE

A similar critical care unit has a standard of 14 HPPD. The unit has the same two acuities — acuity 1, or 24 HPPD, and acuity 2, or 12 HPPD — and a daily fixed HPD of 29.7 hours for indirect nursing care salaries. The unit experienced the same patients and staffing for a specific day.

Sample Calculations

$$\text{Standard} = 14 \text{ HPPD} + 29.7 \text{ fixed hours}$$
$$\text{Standard} \times \text{number of patients} + \text{fixed overhead hours} = \text{total hours required}$$
$$14 \times 11 \text{ Patients} + 29.7 \text{ hours} = 183.7 \text{ hours required}$$

$$\text{Productivity} = \frac{\text{hours required}}{\text{hours worked}} = \frac{183.7}{189.7} = 96\%$$

In this example, the staff was 4% less efficient or productive than the standard required because it utilized 6 hours more than the standard required.

$$189.7 - 183.7 = 6 \text{ hours over standard}$$

3. A third kind of productivity standard is a flat average HPPD figure that includes direct and indirect nursing care.

EXAMPLE

The same critical care unit has a standard of 16 HPPD that includes direct and indirect hours for all patient care services.

Sample Calculations

Standard $\times$ number of patients = required hours
16 HPPD $\times$ 11 patients = 176 hours required

$$\text{Productivity} = \frac{\text{hours required}}{\text{hours worked}} = \frac{176.0}{189.7} = 93\%$$

In this case, the unit was only 93% productive because it actually used 13.7 hours more than the standard required.

189.7 − 176.0 hours = 13.7 hours over standard

The specific standard implemented by a hospital or nursing department should be chosen to fit the individual needs and expertise of the hospital or clinical unit. Examples of productivity standards for other nursing departments are displayed in Table 3-9. A nursing department usually establishes productivity goals within the range of 95% to 105%.

Strategies to Increase Productivity

Improving productivity in health care organizations will depend partly on intensifying the self-disciplined performance of large groups of professionals.[9] Increasing productivity of professional workers involves matching employee characteristics with job characteristics to increase worker satisfaction and motivation. Turnover rates for staff nurses ranged from 37% to 67% percent at the beginning of the current decade.[10] These high rates significantly decrease the productivity of a unit as a result of high orientation and training costs.

Effective support services were identified as a key to increasing nursing productivity in a 1984 study of 10 East Coast hospitals.[11] The study showed that nursing HPPD figures were reduced in institutions that provided effective transportation, dietary, central supply, and pharmacy support. This same study showed essentially no decrease in HPPD nursing standards or increase in productivity as a result of the following factors[11]:

- Skill mix of the nursing staff
- Hospital days of patients over age 65
- Nursing model used to deliver care
- Unit dose medication system

Table 3-9   Nursing Productivity Standards

Unit	Unit of Service (UOS)	Standard	Calculations
Recovery room	Inpatient recoveries	2 hr/UOS	2 hr × recoveries = labor required
	Outpatient recoveries	3 hr/UOS	3 hr × recoveries = labor required

Emergency department	Emergency visits	.5 hr/UOS + 59.4 hr fixed labor	.5 hr × visits + 59.4 hr = labor required
			Fixed labor:
			  Head nurse = 5.7 hr
			  PLN nurse = 5.7 hr
			  2 MICNs/shift = 16 hr × 3 shifts = 48 hr

Medical–surgical unit	Patient days	a. 5.8 HPPD	5.8 HPPD × patients = total labor required for direct and indirect nursing care includes: head nurse, patient care givers, ward secretaries, VP nursing, ADON, off-shift supervisors, etc.
		b. 5 HPPD + 10.8 HPD fixed overhead	5 HPPD × patients + 10.8 HPD fixed = required labor Fixed time includes: Head nurse = 5.7 HPD Allocation of nursing administration over-head = 5.1 HPD
		c. 5 HPPD + 5.7 HPD for head nurse	5 HPPD × patients + 5.7 HPD = required labor

- Number of inpatient beds
- Occupancy rate of hospital

The most recently identified strategy to increase nurse productivity is based on implementing computer support for nursing to reduce a significant amount of the paperwork and documentation that nurses do. Dr. Ralph Korpman has been instrumental in the development of a bedside nursing computer terminal that will significantly increase the productivity of nursing by decreasing documentation time. Dr. Korpman's research shows that 40% of all nursing time is spent filling out forms and meeting documentation requirements.[12] Computerization can significantly reduce the time it takes nurses to do these tasks. Therefore, nursing productivity standards can be reduced and/or productivity increased.

Incentive Plans

The for-profit sector has been successful in increasing productivity by the implementation of incentive programs and plans for managers and employees. The health care industry as a whole has been very reluctant to develop and implement such an approach to productivity.

For-profit multi-hospital systems have begun to implement fiscal incentive programs for their management personnel that include availability of stock-options and profit-sharing programs. Management incentive programs usually include a bonus if the manager's fiscal performance is within specific guidelines. There are strong predictions that the not-for-profit sector will need to develop and implement incentive programs or it will lose top management talent to the for-profit sector because of an inability to compete in terms of compensation programs.

The author has felt for a long time that nursing productivity could be improved if financial incentives could be built into the acuity or patient classification system. It is common knowledge that a nurse is not a nurse is not a nurse. There are nurses who can carry a heavy assignment and deliver excellent patient care, while there are others who cannot handle even a light patient load. Why not reward nurses for their ability to manage and organize varying patient assignments?

No one has quite figured out how to pay nurses by case load, but there is a method to reward a unit or department that is more productive than expected.

EXAMPLE

A 26-bed medical-surgical unit has a productivity standard of 5.8 HPPD. (This HPPD standard includes direct care and indirect care and all nursing overhead.) The average patient census on the unit is 20.

Incentive Plan

The unit has a productivity goal of 5.8 HPPD for total nursing care. The unit will split any savings achieved by being more productive with the hospital on a 50:50 basis. Individual employees will receive quarterly productivity bonuses based on their FTE status in relationship to the whole department.

In a particular quarter, the unit assigned acuities and nurses' assignments in such a manner that it cared for all the patients at an average of 5.0 HPPD. This represented a 0.8 HPPD savings of labor cost for each patient. The unit experienced 420 patient days for the quarter.

Sample Calculations

HPPD savings × patient days = total labor savings

Total labor savings $\times$ average hourly rate = total dollar savings
Total dollar savings $\div$ 2 = incentive pool
Incentive pool $\div$ unit FTEs = productivity bonus/FTE

0.8 HPPD $\times$ 420 patient days = 336 hours saved
336 hours $\times$ \$12/hour = \$4,032 saved
\$4,032 $\div$ 2 = \$2,016
\$2,016 $\div$ 18 bonus FTEs = \$112/FTE

The HPPD savings is multiplied by the number of patient days on the unit, and then the total hours saved is multiplied by the average hourly rate for salaries. The total dollar savings is then divided by 2 to determine the incentive pool that the unit has earned. The unit's incentive pool is divided by the number of FTEs in the unit, and employees receive a quarterly bonus check based on their FTE. When there are no savings or the unit actually utilized more resources than called for by the standard, it is reflected in performance appraisals, and no bonus checks are issued. In this particular case, each full-time employee on the unit received a productivity bonus check for \$112. If an employee is designated a 0.6 FTE, he would receive a check for \$67.20.

Calculations

Bonus/FTE $\times$ FTE = prorated productivity bonus
\$112 $\times$ 0.6 FTE = \$67.20

Quality of patient care would be reviewed and maintained on this unit by the performance appraisal process, the quality assurance program, patient satisfaction survey, and through a peer review process. If staffing was reduced to levels at which medication errors, patient and/or physician dissatisfaction, and complications resulted, appropriate measures would be taken. Goals for these parameters need to be maintained for a unit to receive the productivity bonuses. Incentive programs such as this require strong managerial guidance, monitoring, and intervention. They can allow the institution to be competitive in the marketplace and may be crucial for maintaining talented human resources in the institution.

SUMMARY

In an environment of increased competition and decreasing profit margins for health care services, health care managers and administrators can benefit from the advantages gained from managerial cost accounting and productivity tools. The major concepts presented in this chapter that will assist the nurse manager to function more efficiently to cope with the rapidly changing health care environment include the following:

1. *Total costs* to provide patient care services are composed of

fixed costs and *variable costs*. Fixed costs are the expenses the hospital experiences no matter how many patients need care (*e.g.,* minimum staffing requirements, the overhead of administration and support departments, utilities, etc.). Variable costs are expenses that are experienced by the hospital based on the volume of patients who require services. Examples of variable expenses include staffing by acuity, medical supplies for patient care, linen costs, and so on.

2. In the 1980s inpatient census is consistently declining, making it more significant to monitor and control cost per patient day rather than total expenses. As volume decreases below the break-even point, cost to deliver the service usually increases unless management intervenes.

3. There are two methods of implementing a managerial cost accounting system. Direct costing is the method of accounting for all expenses directly experienced by a department to deliver patient care services. Full costing is the method of accounting for all expenses involved in providing patient care services by transferring or allocating all indirect costs to the patient care units or departments.

4. *Direct costs* are the costs actually incurred in delivering patient care services to the patients. Examples of direct costs include staff nurses' salaries and medical supplies.

   Indirect costs are expenses that are necessary to support the delivery of patient care such as nursing management salaries, expense for the medical records department, hospital administration, financing costs, and so on.

5. The nursing manager of a department can get a better perspective of the total costs to deliver patient care services and the contribution margin of the department when the hospital has implemented a managerial cost-accounting system. When a department manager is responsible for only the direct costs of a patient care department, he or she has a very limited perspective of the fiscal operations of the department.

6. *Break-even analysis* is an evaluation of the cost-volume-profit relationships to deliver patient care services. The break-even patient census in a hospital is the number of patients who, in theory, pay for the average daily expenses of hospital operations. The *safety margin* is the number of patients over the break-even point on which the hospital bases its operating budget. Break-even patients + margin of safety = budgeted patient census.

7. A manager must have an understanding of the following factors that influence hospital:

- Physician practice patterns
- Patient census or occupancy rate
- Productivity
- Group purchasing rates for supplies
- Overutilization of supplies
- Utilization of health and employee benefits
- Hospital programs and services

8. Productivity increases are one of the biggest challenges facing the health care industry in the 1980s. *Productivity* is defined as the measure of the efficiency of the utilization of human resources in the delivery of patient care services. It will be important for hospitals to develop productivity standards for all procedures and all hospital departments.

9. Productivity standards are basically calculated in the following manner:

$$\frac{\text{Hours required}}{\text{Hours actually worked}} = \text{Measure of productivity}$$

10. Methods to increase productivity in nursing include the following:

- Decrease nursing turnover
- Match individual characteristics to job characteristics for a better job "fit"
- Implement effective support departments to assist nursing with non-nursing tasks (*e.g.*, transport teams, dietary aides, central supply systems, etc.)
- Implement computer systems to decrease the paperwork and documentation for nursing

REFERENCES

1. Managerial Cost Accounting. Chicago, IL, American Hospital Association, 1980
2. Walker DD: The cost of nursing care in hospitals. JONA 13(3):3-18
3. Harju M, Sabatino F: Productivity efforts on the rise. Hospitals p 89, November 1984
4. Mistarz J: Cost-accounting: A solution, but a problem. Hospitals p 96, October 1984
5. Poulsen G: Detailed costing system nets efficiency, savings. Hospitals p 106, October 1984
6. Staley M, Luciano K: Eight steps to costing nursing services. Nurs Management p 35, October 1984

7. Kendrick JW: Understanding Productivity: An Introduction to the Dynamics of Productivity Change, p 1. Baltimore, Johns Hopkins, 1977
8. Bermas N, Van Slyck A: Patient classification systems and the nursing department. Hospitals p 99, November 1984
9. Guthrie M, Maver G, Zawacki R, Cougar JD: Productivity: How much does this job mean? Nurs Management 16(2):19, 1985
10. Friss LO: Work force policy perspectives: Registered nurses. J Health Politics Policy Law 5(4), 1981
11. Swenson B, Wolfe H, Schroeder R: Effectively employing support services: The key for increasing nursing personnel productivity. Modern Healthcare p 101, December 1984
12. Korpman R: Patient care information systems: Looking to the future, Part Two. Software in Healthcare p 27, June-July 1984

ADDITIONAL READINGS

1. Computers in Nursing. Philadelphia, JB Lippincott, March-April 1985
2. Horngren C: Cost Accounting: A Managerial Emphasis, 2nd ed. Englewood Cliffs, NJ, Prentice-Hall, 1967
3. Korpman R: Patient care information systems. Parts I, III, IV. Software in Healthcare April-May, August-September, October-November 1984
4. Hoffman FM: Financial Management for Nurse Managers. Norwalk, CT, Appleton-Century-Crofts, 1984
5. Esmond TH: Budgeting Procedures for Hospitals. Chicago, American Hospital Association, 1982
6. Althaus JH, Hardyck NMcD, Pierce PB, Rodgers MS: Decentralized budgeting: Holding the pursestrings, Part 2. JONA 12(6):34-38, 1982
7. Higgerson NJ, Van Slyke A: Variable billing for services: New fiscal direction for nursing. JONA 12(6):20-27, 1982

Budgeting for Nursing Managers

A BUDGET can be defined as the annual statement or process of identifying probable revenues and expenditures for the organization. A budget is viewed by some as an "educated guess" regarding the volume of goods and/or services the organization will deliver the next year, as well as the expenses required to deliver those goods and/or services. Budgeting can be considered the process by which decision makers allocate resources to support particular programs that attain the strategic plan of the organization for the coming year.[1] The budget is used as a master plan for annual operations, as a control mechanism, and as an evaluation tool to determine the organization's performance over the past year.[2]

Nursing managers and administrators have frequently been "handed" their budgets in the past, without actually providing any input or rationale for the actual figures identified. This is one of the most important reasons nursing has been reluctant to assume financial responsibility for budgeting functions in the past. Another significant reason is rooted in the lack of financial courses in traditional bachelor's and master's programs in nursing to prepare nurse managers to assume this responsibility.

It must be acknowledged that there are many health care institutions that do involve their nurse managers in all phases of the budgeting process. In the past, these organizations have been in the minority, however. This trend is rapidly changing. Administrators are becoming aware of the fact that nurse managers on the unit level can best identify the trends in patient census and acuity that are likely to occur in the future. The department manager can accomplish these projections in the most efficient manner because he or she is closer to the actual day-to-day operations, efficiencies, and inefficiencies.

This is the major reason a chapter on budgeting is included in this text. Nurse managers at all levels of the organization need skills in the development, management, and evaluation of a budget to be successful professionally, as well as to assist their organization to survive and prosper.

This chapter will focus on basic budgeting terminology, functions of the budget, the processes of developing, managing, and revising the budget, and evaluation of financial performance by means of the variance report. It is important to note that every organization has a different budgeting process with varying methods of actually calculating revenues and expenses, different forms to complete, and different methods of submitting and approving budgets. This chapter will outline a generic process and include the most common procedures for health care institutions.

At this point it is important to note that the annual operational budget should, ideally, be based on the organization's well-thought-out strategic plan. The *strategic plan* identifies the goals the organization wants to accomplish in the next 3 to 5 years.[3] The annual operational or short-range plan consists of the goals and objectives the organization will accomplish each year. The operational or annual budget is the method by which the institution plans to accomplish these goals financially. The strategic planning process is described in greater detail in Chapter 6. This chapter focuses on developing a budget to accomplish the annual goals and objectives of the organization.

OBJECTIVES

Upon completing this chapter, the reader will be able to

1. Outline the basic process of budgeting in a health care institution.

2. Understand basic budgeting terminology.

3. Understand the use and rationale for a position control form.

4. Outline the basic concepts in zero-based budgeting, program planning and budgeting, and management by objectives.

5. Evaluate historical data to project future revenue and/or units of service volume for a department.

6. Identify and calculate fixed costs and/or overhead for a nursing department.

7. Identify and calculate the variable costs to deliver health care services.

8. Identify the components of the variance report and explain specific variations between budgeted and actual figures.

9. Identify and implement specific strategies to manage a budget for a unit in a productive manner.

10. Identify the differences between flexible and nonflexible budgets and variance systems.

11. Differentiate between productive and nonproductive time and be able to budget for both kinds of expenses.

12. Understand the basic process of capital equipment budgeting.

13. Define the rationale and importance of developing a cash budget.

BUDGET METHODS

There are approximately four different budgeting methods that organizations have used to develop their annual operating budgets. These four methods will be outlined individually; they include the following:

1. Flat percentage increase
2. Planning, programming, and budgeting (PPB)
3. Management by objectives (MBO)
4. Zero-based budgeting (ZBB)

Each of these methods has appeared in the budgeting protocols of hospitals in the past and should be understood by the nurse manager. Most hospitals use a combination of one or more of these methods in their actual budget preparation.

The *flat percentage increase method* is the simplest method for departmental budgeting and has been commonly used in hospitals in the past. The upcoming budget for a department is very easily developed by annualizing the current year-to-date expenses and multiplying those figures by a certain percentage. The most commonly used figure is the inflation rate or the consumer price index (CPI).

SAMPLE CALCULATIONS

Salary expense Y-T-D $\times$ annualizing figure = annualized salary expense
Annualized salary expense $\times$ inflation factor = budgeted salaries for next year
$450,00 $\times$ 1.7 = $765,000
(salaries/7 months)
$765,000 $\times$ 1.12 = $866,800
(12% inflation)

Budgeting by this method is simple and quick and does not require a lot of time, resources or thought to produce. The weaknesses of the method include the following:

- It does not deal with issues of productivity and efficiency.
- Expenses can escalate drastically on an annual basis.

The second method, *planning, programming, and budgeting,* or *PPB,* was introduced by President Johnson in 1965.[4] PPB lasted for only about six years as a formal method of budgeting in the federal government. However, the principles of PPB live on in many private and public organizations. The most important budgeting principle that came from the PPB system is the development of objectives to determine which programs and/or services are financially supported by the organization by being included in the budget. The steps in the PPB budget process include the following:

1. Development of departmental objectives and goals
2. Evaluation of each program and service to meet those objectives, including a cost-benefit analysis
3. Examination of alternative programs and/or services to meet the objectives
4. Development of the budget based on the analysis of the alternative programs and/or services to meet the objectives and financial limitations present

Management by objectives, or *MBO,* was originated by Peter Drucker in the 1950s. In 1973 MBO was introduced into the federal budget process after Drucker popularized the process in conjunction with George Odiorne.[5,6] MBO is very similar to PPB, but it requires less financial analysis of alternative programs and/or services to accomplish the organization's objectives. MBO is the process of supporting programs and services and including them in the budget if they assist the organization reach its predetermined objectives.

Zero-based budgeting, or *ZBB,* is the final budget method that will be discussed. ZBB was first developed by Peter Pyhrr at Texas Instruments in the 1970s.[4] Jimmy Carter first applied ZBB in the government when he was governor of Georgia.

ZBB emphasizes management's responsibility for the planning, budgeting, and evaluation functions of the organization's resources. ZBB includes an analysis of alternative programs and services on three different levels: the minimum objective level, the current objective level, and the improvement objective level. It places new programs on an equal footing with existing programs by requiring a ranking of program priorities and thereby provides a systematic basis for allocating resources by means of the budgeting process.

BUDGET FUNCTIONS

The budget ideally serves or operationalizes three major management functions: the planning function, the management of ongoing activities, and the control of spending. When the budget process acknowledges these three functions and implements them in the process of developing the budget, the organization will receive maximum benefits from its available resources.

The planning function is implemented through the budget process when resources are allocated to objectives identified in the organization's strategic plan. When an organization develops a budget that does not coincide with a long-range or strategic plan, its resources will not be utilized in the most efficient manner.

According to Shillinglaw and associates, the budgetary planning function has six major objectives[7]:

1. To force managers to analyze the company's activities for appropriateness

2. To direct management's attention from the present to the future

3. To enable management to anticipate problems or opportunities in time to deal with them

4. To reinforce managers' motivation to work to achieve the company's objectives

5. To remind managers of the actions they have decided upon

6. To provide a reference point for control reporting

The budget process is a series of vertical and horizontal communications among managers in the organization to develop a set of integrated and realizable objectives and financial support consistent with the organization's mission statement.[7]

The management of ongoing activities is accomplished when managers compare actual expenditures with budgeted figures and make adjustments to operations to maintain their fiscal goals.

The control of spending is accomplished through the budget by means of monthly and year-to-date variance reports that compare budgeted with actual expenses. Managers are usually evaluated based on their financial performance and budget adherence. It is this factor that allows the budget to actualize the control of the spending function.

In summary, Table 4-1 outlines the major budget functions and characteristics of each function as it relates to the budget process.

Table 4-1 Functions of the Budget and Their Characteristics

Budget Function	Goal	Time Sequence	Responsibility
Planning	Determination of objectives	Budget preparation	Top administration
Management of activities	Identify programs to meet objectives	Entire budget cycle	Top administration and department directors
Control of spending	Hold managers accountable to implement programs within fiscal guidelines established	Execution and audit stages of budget	Top administration and department directors

BASIC BUDGETING

As previously mentioned, the budget is an "educated guess" about the business or revenue for an organization for the next year, coupled with the expenses the organization will experience. In a health care institution, the business is determined by the number of health care services the institution believes it will deliver to the community in the upcoming year. The business volume the health care institution delivers is categorized by the broad term *units of service*. A unit of service is the specific unit of health care service a department delivers to its customers. For example, in an acute care institution the unit of service is the *patient day*. Inpatient stays are calculated based on the days a patient is hospitalized. Therefore, the unit of inpatient health care service is patient days.

On the other hand, the unit of service for an outpatient kidney dialysis unit is usually considered a dialysis treatment. The units of service in the inpatient surgery department could be defined as major surgeries, minor surgeries, or the average time for all surgeries (*e.g.*, 3 hours of surgery equals one unit of surgery service [UOS]). A more detailed list of various units of services for different departments in an acute care hospital is included in Table 4-2.

Units of service are projected for the upcoming year based on the number of units of service the department delivered over the past year, adjusted to reflect the increases or decreases expected to occur in the future. The increases or decreases are greatly influenced by the results of the environmental assess-

Table 4-2   Units of Service for Hospital Departments

Department	Unit of Service
Nursing	Patient day
Surgery	Minor procedures
	Major procedures
	Average time for all procedures
Outpatient dialysis	Dialysis procedures
Laboratory	CAP units
Dietary	Meals served
Emergency department	Patient visits
Maintenance department	Work orders

ment the top management team does in the process of developing the strategic plan. After the units of service are identified, the projected departmental revenues can be calculated. Revenues are calculated by multiplying projected units of service by the average charges for a particular unit of service. An inpatient medical-surgical nursing unit could calculate projected patient revenues by multiplying the average daily room charge by the number of patient days budgeted. It must be mentioned that this is a very simplified method of projecting patient revenues. The actual revenue that the institution will receive is affected by a number of other factors resulting from the prospective reimbursement environment and other factors.

SAMPLE CALCULATIONS

Budgeted patient days × room charge = projected revenue

12,000 × $300 = $3,600,000

After projected revenues are calculated, expenditures to deliver the service are calculated. Health care organizations are labor intensive because of their focus on service. Salaries constitute 50% to 70% of total expenditures in the budget. Other expenditures in a health care setting include employee benefits, depreciation, administration, legal fees, medical and nonmedical supplies, maintenance, daily operation of plant, physician compensation, and so on.

When expenses are subtracted from revenues, projected profits remain. When those profits are found to be too small, management returns to the "drawing board" to reduce expenses.

After a budget is implemented, it is monitored on an ongoing basis by comparing actual figures with budgeted figures. These comparisons of budgeted figures with actual figures are usually done on a pay-period basis, monthly basis, quarterly basis, and a year-to-date basis.[8] There are 26 pay periods, 12 months, and four quarters in a fiscal year. Institutions usually develop monthly financial reports that exhibit monthly, quarterly, and year-to-date figures to evaluate how well they are approximating their budget figures. For the institution with a fiscal year beginning in October, quarterly reports cover these respective months:

EXAMPLE OF OCTOBER FISCAL YEAR

Quarter	Months
First quarter	October, November, December
Second quarter	January, February, March
Third quarter	April, May, June
Fourth quarter	July, August, September

Year-to-date (y-t-d) figures represent the total of all actual figures from the beginning of the fiscal year to the date of the specific report.

Budgeted figures are the numbers the institution projects for revenue and expenses based on their "educated guessing" before the actual fact. *Actual figures* are the exact expenses and revenues the institution experienced. The difference between budgeted and actual figures is called the *variance*. The *variance report* is a report that compares the budgeted figures with the actual figures and calculates the difference. Large differences usually require some sort of explanation and/or justification from the accountable manager. (The variance report will be discussed in greater detail later in this chapter.)

POSITION CONTROL

The *position control* is the list of approved labor positions for the department. The position control displays the approved positions by category of personnel (*e.g.,* RN, LVN, or aide, as well as by the number of full-time equivalents [FTEs]). An FTE is a full-time position that can be equated to 40 hours of work per week. By definition, a full-time position or equivalent works 40 hours per week or 80 hours per pay period.

An FTE is a time equivalent of 2,080 paid hours per year (40 hours per week x 52 weeks = 2,080 hours per year). This 2,080 hours per year includes all paid hours for an FTE. Paid hours include actually worked time, or *productive time,* as well as *nonproductive time,* or vacation time, sick time, education time, and so on. An FTE is not a person or a job. It is a unit of time that is approved by administration for pay or compensation to do a particular job. Table 4-3 shows a sample position control sheet.

This sample position control shows that the unit has filled one of its RN positions with an LVN, because it is over on LVNs and under on RN positions. Overall, the unit could hire an additional .2 FTE of a ward secretary. This .2 FTE could be filled by a currently employed part-time secretary working 1 additional day per week or by a per diem secretary working only 1 day a week.

An FTE always equals 40 hours of work per week or 80 hours of work per pay period. With the increased popularity of flexible and creative staffing patterns and work weeks, a full-time employee at a particular institution may not be equivalent to a 1 FTE.

For example, if an institution has the 12-hour-shift option, and its full-time employees work three 12-hour-shifts a week, each 12-hour-shift employee is actually only a .9 FTE.

SAMPLE CALCULATIONS

Hours/day × days worked = hours/week ÷ 40 hours/FTE = number of FTEs
12 hours × 3 days = 36 hours/week ÷ 40 hours = .9 FTE

Table 4-3   Sample Position Control

Positions	Full-Time Equivalents		
	Approved	*Filled*	*Status*
Department director	1.0	1.0	0
Registered nurses	6.4	5.4	−1.0
Licensed vocational nurses	4.0	5.0	+1.0
Ward secretaries	2.2	2.0	−.2
Total positions	13.6	13.4	−.2

Similarly, if a regular 8-hour-shift employee works 3 days a week, he or she is a .6 FTE.

CALCULATIONS

Hours/day $\times$ days worked = hours/week $\div$ 40 hours/FTE = number of FTEs
8 hours $\times$ 3 days = 24 hours/week $\div$ 40 hours = .6 FTE

The hours for an FTE vary with the unit of time being considered. Suppose that in a 2-week period a nurse manager experiences 160 hours of overtime on her unit. She wants to calculate how many FTEs of additional per diem nurses to hire to eliminate the cost of overtime. Remember that 1 FTE in a pay period equals 80 hours of time worked. Therefore,

---

SAMPLE CALCULATIONS

160 Overtime hours in a pay period $\div$ 80 hours/FTE = 2 FTEs

---

The head nurse would need two additional FTEs who each work 40 hours per week or 80 hours per pay period to eliminate the need to ask other staff to work overtime to care for the patients.

As previously mentioned, an FTE equals 2,080 hours of productive and nonproductive time on an annual basis. The hospital will pay an FTE for 2,080 hours, but not all of that time is paid-for time actually worked. Some of those 2,080 hours are considered benefit or nonproductive time. *Benefit or nonproductive time* is the time the institution pays the employee for actually not working. Benefit time includes holiday time, vacation time, sick time, personal time off (PTO), and so on. The actual amount of time for each employee is determined by the individual organization's benefit policies.

For budgeting purposes, this benefit time must be calculated as an expense for the department. It must also be subtracted from the actual productive time available to care for patients. For example, if an institution pays a full-time employee for 2 weeks of vacation, 8 holidays, and 10 sick days a year, that employee can actually care for patients only 1,856 hours per year instead of the full 2,080 hours per year.

SAMPLE CALCULATIONS

---

2 Weeks' vacation = 80 hours
10 Sick days = 80 hours
8 Holidays = 64 hours
Total benefit time = 224 hours
2,080 Hours − 224 hours = 1,856 hours of productive time available for patient care

---

Labor costs or salary costs are divided into fixed and variable costs. *Fixed labor costs* are paid no matter what the activity or patient volume on a unit. For example, on an inpatient nursing unit, fixed labor costs include the nursing manager, unit secretary, clinical specialist, and any other role that does not vary or flex with the number of patients on the unit. In most institutions, this represents the nursing department director or head nurse, who is primarily responsible for the management of the unit or department. Other positions that may be considered as fixed time because they do not flex with patient volume or acuity include the following:

- Monitor technicians on a telemetry or critical care unit
- Unit secretary
- Clinical specialist
- Unit aide or orderly

Variable time, or *labor costs,* on the other hand, are the budgeted positions and time that flex or vary with specific patient census and/or acuity. *Acuity* is a measure of the nursing resources that are required to care for a particular patient. *Acuity systems* enable the nurse manager to categorize patients based on their individual needs for nursing care. By identifying and categorizing patient needs, the manager can schedule the appropriate skill level and number of nurses to care for those patients. On the budget, the expenses for variable time are expected to increase or decrease based on the actual units of service and patient acuity the department or unit experiences.

Fixed costs are the expenses or costs that a department experiences for daily operations irrespective of volume. Fixed costs include the cost of fixed time (previously discussed), lights, electricity, interest expense, depreciation, telephone service, unit supplies, housekeeping, and so on. *Variable costs,* on the other hand, are the expenses that are incurred as a direct result of a specific volume of patients. Examples of variable costs include medical supplies, nonmedical supplies (patient and forms), direct care givers (nursing staff), meals, and so on. (These concepts were described in greater detail in Chapter 3.)

THE BUDGET PROCESS

There are as many budget processes and procedures as there are organizations. The writer will therefore outline and define a fairly simple generic process that focuses on the whats and the whys of budgeting rather than on the specific forms and procedures used. The budget process contains the following major steps[9]:

1. Environmental assessment
2. Statement of mission and objectives
3. Assumptions about the future
4. Setting operational objectives
5. Preparation of budget manuals
6. Preparation of project packages
7. Completion of departmental budgets
8. Departmental budget hearings
9. Presentation of institutional budget to finance committee
10. Implementation of operational budget
11. Analysis of budget variances
12. Year-end evaluation and environmental assessment

Step 1: The Environmental Assessment

Environmental assessment is the process of analyzing the operating environment of the specific health care institution. Before setting future goals and objectives, it is vital for an organization to have a clear understanding of its current position and the kind of environment in which it is operating. The following are specific items that are included in an environmental assessment:

- The current strengths and weaknesses of the institution
- The characteristics of the external environment (*e.g.,* increased competition, increasing population, payor classifications, and changing socioeconomic factors in the community

- The current role the institution plays within the health care delivery system of the community

(The topic of environmental assessment is dealt with in greater detail in Chapter 6.)

Step 2: Statement of the Institution's Mission and Objectives

The institution's mission statement is the broad statement of its primary purpose for existence. It is important for the budgeting process to review, clarify, and/or revise this mission statement annually based on a changing environment. For example, a community hospital has a mission statement, "Dedicated to providing services to meet the total health care needs of the community."

As technology increases, the institution will need to decide if it is reasonable and even possible to supply all health care services to a community regardless of the cost, volume, and demand. The hospital may decide that it needs to revise its mission statement to reflect a more reasonable position. Budgets are designed to be a financial reflection of the organization's goals and objectives, and so it is important that these items are kept current and constitute a shared commitment for the entire organization.

Institutional objectives are broad goals of the organization that flow from the mission statement. Examples of institutional objectives include the following:

1. To provide care to patients regardless of their ability to pay
2. To provide the community with the needed health care services directly or indirectly through referral to appropriate agencies
3. To provide an acceptable level of quality services at the least possible cost

These broad objectives are key issues in determining which programs and services are included in the operational budget. They determine the level of expenses that are acceptable and the pricing mechanisms that determine revenue projections.

The institution's mission statement and broad general objectives typically remain constant from one year to another. However, in a rapidly changing health care environment of the mid-1980s, many institutions may have to rethink their mission statements and possibly redefine them. Institutions that focus only on the care of acute inpatients may have severe problems surviving and maintaining a leadership position in the industry.

Step 3: Identifying Assumptions About the Future

Step 3 can be accomplished by use of the management tool of scenario building. This management tool has recently become popular in the health care industry and is utilized primarily by futurists. *Scenario building* is writing a story about what could possibly happen in the future after identifying driving trends in the environment.[10]

Step 4: Setting Operational Objectives

Step 4 includes the development of departmental goals for the coming year. Departmental goals should coincide with the larger, broader objectives of the organization.

EXAMPLE

An institution has the following organizational objective:
Organizational objective: To provide an acceptable level of quality services at the least possible cost.
An example of an annual objective for a surgery department that fits in with this organizational objective could be the following:
Surgery annual objective: Develop a low-cost same-day surgery program by October 15, 19x1 as exhibited by the scheduling of the first procedure.

It is important that annual departmental objectives match the general organizational objectives for the organization to be effective and efficient in meeting its objectives.

Step 5: Preparation of Budget Manuals

Preparation of budget manuals is the responsibility of the finance department and the CFO, and involves the development of the budget forms, timeliness, and expectations for the department directors in preparing their budgets. Budget policies, procedures, forms, and actual methods of calculating budgets vary considerably from one organization to another. Components of most budget packets include the following:

1. Instructions for completing budget forms and making calculations
2. Sample budget calculations

3. Approved position control sheet
4. Blank budget forms
5. Blank spreadsheet
6. Capital equipment request forms
7. Departmental objective forms

Step 6: Preparation of Projection Packages

Step 6 involves the identification of future volume projections for the different services and products the institution provides. For a nursing department, this translates into identifying the number of patient days the hospital will experience during the coming year. These projections are usually identified by revising current year-to-date patient days up or down based on the organization's assumptions about the future. The CFO is responsible for this step in collaboration with the administrator and individual department directors. Table 4-4 is a sample worksheet for forecasting units of service for a nursing unit. The forecasting procedure includes a comparison of the current budgeted and actual patient days experienced and a preliminary projection of the next year's volume. The final column of

Table 4-4   Worksheet for Forecasting Units of Service

Year _____
Department _____
Prepared by _____

Month	Current Year Budget	Current Year Actual	Preliminary Projection	Approved Units
Oct	820	980	950	950
Nov	810	850	850	850
Dec	800	780	750	750
Jan	880	850	800	800
Feb	790	800	780	780
Mar	880	900	880	880
Apr	820	800	780	780
May	870	(870)	880	880
Jun	850	(850)	840	840
Jul	860	(860)	850	850
Aug	900	(900)	880	880
Sep	800	(800)	820	820
Total	10,080	10,240	10,060	10,060
% Change		+1.5%	−1.7%	−1.7%

Comments:_____

_____

_____

the worksheet consists of the approved units of service for the next year's budget.

Step 7: Completion of Departmental Budgets

Completion of departmental budgets is the step that most department managers dread on an annual basis. After receiving their projected service volume for the next year, department managers are responsible for calculating their annual expense budgets.

The largest line item on any expense budget in a health care institution is for salaries. Some institutions calculate their budgets based on the average hourly cost for their employees. Other institutions calculate their salary budgets using actual employee salaries. The level of detail or sophistication in calculating an expense budget is usually determined by the CFO or administrator's attention to detail. Remember that a budget is just an "educated guess," and the more detailed it is, the more time and money are required to develop it. There is a definite cost attached to being very precise in budgets. If an institution calculates salary expense based on actual salaries, as soon as someone quits, the budget becomes inaccurate. Therefore, the cost of developing budget detail must be considered when identifying the specific budget process for an organization.

SALARY EXPENSE

Salary expense for a health care organization includes these components:

- Productive time or time actually worked
- Nonproductive time or benefit time

Nonproductive time is time the hospital pays employees for vacations, sick time, holiday time, personal time, education time, and orientation time. Many hospital managers are unaware of the extensive costs associated with these nonproductive hours for which employees are reimbursed. Efficient health care management includes close attention to the management of nonproductive time, as well as productive time.

Productive salaries in nursing can be divided into direct patient care and indirect patient care. *Direct patient care* salary costs account for the nursing salaries of direct care givers at the bedside. *Indirect patient care* salary costs include the cost for unit management, unit secretaries, monitor technicians, director of nursing, staffing office secretaries, off-shift supervision, and so on.

A simple method of calculating salary expense for a nursing unit with a standard of 5 HPPD for total direct and indirect nursing care follows:

SAMPLE CALCULATIONS

Projected patient days = 12,000
Nursing care standard = 5 hours per patient day
Patient days × standard = total productive hours required
12,000 × 5 HPPD = 60,000 total hours required for patient care
60,00 Total care hours
÷ 2,080 productive hours/FTE = 28.8 productive FTEs
28.8 FTEs × 1.15 (benefit time = 15%/FTE) = 33.1 total FTEs
33.1 FTEs = total productive and nonproductive FTE's required
33.1 FTEs
× 2,080 hours (annual hours/FTE)
× $14/hour = $963,872 annual salary expense

The total salary expense to care for 12,000 patient days, giving each patient 5 hours of care per day at an average hourly salary of $14/hour is $963,872. This total salary expense includes direct and indirect patient care costs because the nursing standard of 5 hours per patient day is the total care hours provided the patient in a 24-hour period and includes all roles on the nursing unit, including the following:

- Direct care givers: registered nurses, LVNs, aides
- Indirect care givers: ward secretaries, department manager/head nurse

EMPLOYEE BENEFITS

Employee benefits follow salaries on the expense budget. Employee benefits include the expense for health care insurance and workmen's compensation. The expense is usually charged to each department by allocating a percentage of the institution's total expense for those items based on the number of FTEs in each department.[11]

SAMPLE CALCULATIONS

Total hospital expense for benefits
÷ hospital FTEs = expense/FTE

Expense/FTE $\times$ department's number of FTEs = department's allocation for employee benefits
$1,000,000 ÷ 600 FTEs = $1,667/FTE
$1,667. $\times$ 20 FTEs = $33,340 or department's allocation for benefits

---

Employee benefits are very costly to the organization because of their pure overhead nature. If poorly managed, the expense the organization experiences for workmen's compensation and health care benefits can make a significant dent in the already narrow profit margin of the health care institution. Anything a hospital can do to reduce these liabilities is usually well worth the effort.

BUDGETING FOR SUPPLIES

The second most significant component in the hospital budget is supplies. Barkholz comments that "when labor costs are under control, supply buying and distribution becomes the focal point of a hospital's cost-containment efforts."[12] Hospitals are aggressively seeking out relationships with larger organizations to benefit from group purchasing rates of medical and nonmedical supplies. Hospitals that are experiencing census declines are especially concerned with access to lower group purchasing rates, and this is the major reason smaller institutions are joining with larger multi-hospital organizations.

The majority of health care organizations budget for supplies on a "historical-plus-inflation basis." This method takes last year's actual expense for a category of supplies and divides the annual expense by the year's number of service units to determine cost per unit of service. The cost per unit of service for a commodity is then multiplied by the projected units of service for the next year, and then the total amount is multiplied by a preestablished inflation factor.

For example, an organization has a fiscal year that begins in October, and budget preparation begins in May. The hospital uses its April year-to-date figures for medical supplies (or any other supplies, for that matter) and multiplies them by 1.7 to obtain annualized actual figures. *Annualized figures* are year-to-date actual figures that are manipulated arithmetically to approximate what actual year-end figures are expected to be. Annualized budget figures can be obtained by multiplying year-to-date figures for the first 7 months by 1.7.

SAMPLE CALCULATIONS

Actual cost of medical supplies for first 7 months × 1.7 = annualized cost of medical supplies

$$\$18,000 \times 1.7 = \$30,600$$

If a medical-surgical head nurse experiences medical supply costs of $18,000 from October to the end of April, and the preestablished inflation factor for the coming year is 5%, the head nurse could determine the 19 × 2 budget for medical supplies in the following manner:

SAMPLE CALCULATIONS

Actual cost for first 7 months × Annualizing factor = Annualized medical supply costs

$$\$18,000 \times 1.7 = \$30,600$$

Annualized medical supply costs cost/UOS ÷ annualized UOS = cost of medical supplies/UOS

$$\$30,600 \div 9,600 = \$3.19$$

Medical supply cost/UOS × 19 x 2 UOS × inflation factor = 19 x 2 medical supply budget

$$\$3.19 \times 11,000 \times 1.05 = \$36,815$$

This unit experienced $18,000 in actual medical supply costs for 7 months in 19 × 1. This actual figure was multiplied by 1.7 to determine the annualized cost of medical supplies for the unit of $36,815. The annualized cost of medical supplies is then divided by the annualized units of service or patient days the unit will experience for the entire year to calculate the average cost of medical supplies per patient day. (Patient days can be annualized in the same manner as medical supplies.)

The cost of medical supplies per patient day is then multiplied by the budgeted number of patient days for year 19 × 2 or 11,000 and then by the preestablished inflation factor of 1.05. These calculations result in the budget figure for medical supplies for the unit's 19 × 2 budget. This methodology can also be used to budget for nonmedical supplies, linen, dietary, and maintenance services for a department. It should be emphasized, however, that the method builds in and supports past inefficiencies. If a department experiences excessive costs, excessive utilization of supplies, and/or waste, this methodology promotes the continuance of these practices.

If a manager is concerned with this fact, it is helpful to contact other managers of similar departments at other institutions to compare supply costs per unit of service. It is possible to identify methods and/or potential decreases in supply costs when comparing costs with other organizations. After implementing cost-effective strategies successfully, further budgeting for supplies by this method can be more effective and appropriate. The sample Supply Budget Worksheet could be used to develop a department's annual supply budget.

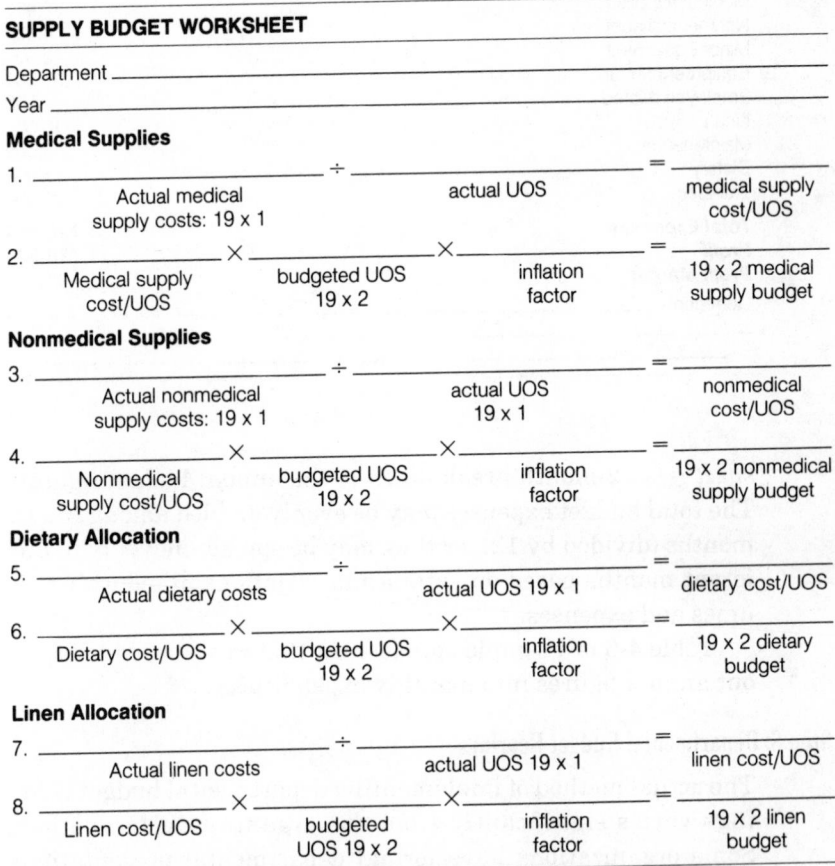

SUPPLY BUDGET WORKSHEET

Department _____

Year _____

Medical Supplies

1. _____ ÷ _____ = _____
   Actual medical supply costs: 19 x 1 / actual UOS / medical supply cost/UOS

2. _____ × _____ × _____ = _____
   Medical supply cost/UOS / budgeted UOS 19 x 2 / inflation factor / 19 x 2 medical supply budget

Nonmedical Supplies

3. _____ ÷ _____ = _____
   Actual nonmedical supply costs: 19 x 1 / actual UOS 19 x 1 / nonmedical cost/UOS

4. _____ × _____ × _____ = _____
   Nonmedical supply cost/UOS / budgeted UOS 19 x 2 / inflation factor / 19 x 2 nonmedical supply budget

Dietary Allocation

5. _____ ÷ _____ = _____
   Actual dietary costs / actual UOS 19 x 1 / dietary cost/UOS

6. _____ × _____ × _____ = _____
   Dietary cost/UOS / budgeted UOS 19 x 2 / inflation factor / 19 x 2 dietary budget

Linen Allocation

7. _____ ÷ _____ = _____
   Actual linen costs / actual UOS 19 x 1 / linen cost/UOS

8. _____ × _____ × _____ = _____
   Linen cost/UOS / budgeted UOS 19 x 2 / inflation factor / 19 x 2 linen budget

The remaining budgetary line items are budgeted for in many different ways by individual organizations. Actual budget figures are established by the CFO based on historical issues and future predictions. Table 4-5 is the sample Departmental Budget Worksheet completed.

After the departmental budget worksheet is completed, the figures are transcribed onto a 12-month spreadsheet. A *spread-*

Table 4-5   Departmental Budget

Patient days	*11,000*
Revenue	*$2,900,000*
Expenses	
Productive salaries	650,000
Nonproductive salaries	120,000
Total salaries	770,000
Employee benefits	100,000
Medical supplies	32,455
Nonmedical supplies	8,000
Minor equipment	2,000
Equipment rental	500
Employee related	500
Linen	10,000
Maintenance	5,000
Dietary	11,000
Transfers	20,000
Total Expenses	*$1,729,455*
Profit	*$1,170,545*
Profit Margin	*40%*
Comments: _____	

sheet is a 12-month break-down of the annual budget figures. The total budget expenses may be evenly divided among the 12 months (divided by 12), or they may be spread unevenly in different months based on significant variations in monthly volumes and expenses.

Table 4-6 is a sample spreadsheet that can be used to break out annual figures into monthly expenditures.

Step 8: Departmental Budget Hearings

The actual method of implementing departmental budget hearings varies significantly from one organization to another. Some organizations have formal departmental presentations before the top administrative officers, whereas other organizations are less formal and have department directors simply present their written budgets to their administrative officer. The formal method of budget presentations or hearings frequently incorporates a review of last year's goals attained, budget performance, as well as a presentation of future departmental goals, objectives, and the budget. Although this process is time-consuming and costly to implement, it gives the depart-

Table 4-6 Sample Departmental Budget Spreadsheet

	Sept	Oct	Nov	Dec	Jan	Feb	Mar	Apr	May	Jun	Jul
UOS											
Revenue											
Expenses											
Productive Salaries											
Nonproductive salaries											
Total salaries											
Benefits											
Medical supplies											
Nonmedical supplies											
Equipment											
Rental											
Employee related expenses											
Linen											
Maintenance											
Dietary											
Transportation											
Total Expenses											
% Profit											
Revenue/UOS											
Expense/UOS											

ment directors an opportunity to receive recognition for their past achievements and performance in the company of the top management team. In many organizations, the time and cost of official budget hearings are considered well worth the cost.

Step 9: Presentation of the Formal Budget to the Finance Committee

After the administrative staff accept the individual departmental budgets, the CFO combines all the departmental budgets into an integrated hospital budget. The institutional budget is then presented formally to the finance committee of the board of directors. This formal presentation usually occurs at the finance committee meeting, which is convened 2 to 3 months prior to the start of the new fiscal year. This 2 to 3 months' lead time allows for the time to make revisions on the suggestions by the finance committee. The budget is then brought back to the committee for approval before the fiscal year begins.

Step 10: Implementation of the Operational Budget

The actual implementation of the operational budget occurs automatically at the beginning of the fiscal year.

Step 11: Monthly Analysis of Budget Variances

The control function of the budget process is accomplished through the ongoing monthly analysis of the actual revenue and expense reports compared with budgeted revenue and expense figures. By comparing actual and budgeted figures and analyzing variances, managers can make the necessary adjustments to operations to meet the organization's financial goals.

Table 4-7 is a sample variance report for a nursing unit.

Managing the Variance. After calculating and analyzing the variance report, managers are responsible for making adjustments to departmental operations to keep expenses in line with revenues and/or service volumes delivered. Nursing management strategies to maintain expenses within predetermined financial goals include the following:

- Reduce overtime expenses.
- Reduce sick-time expenditures.
- Prevent costly expenses for repair of equipment.

Table 4-7   Monthly Variance Report

	Current Month			Year-to-Date		
	Budget	*Actual*	*Variance*	*Budget*	*Actual*	*Variance*
Revenue	**$230,000**	**$229,300**	**(99%)**	**1,700,000**	**1,600,000**	**(94%)**
Patient days	807	822	102%	6028	5795	(96%)
Revenue/UOS	285	278	(98%)	282	276	(97%)
Expense/UOS	101	102	100%	83	83	100%
Expenses						
Salaries	$76,100	$78,000	(102%)	$450,000	$435,000	96%
Medical supplies	700	500	71%	5,500	3,500	63%
Nonmedical supplies	250	400	(160%)	5,700	4,700	82%
Purchased services	150	400	(375%)	3,700	2,900	78%
Maintenance	250	200	80%	5,000	3,000	60%
Equipment rental	0	100	—	500	400	80%
Employee-related expenses	100	200	(200%)	450	500	(111%)
Transfers	3,900	4,500	(115%)	28,000	32,000	(114%)
Other	75	50	67%	650	1,000	(154%)
Total expenses	**81,525**	**84,350**	**(103%)**	**499,500**	**483,000**	**97%**

Explanations: _____

_____

_____

- Utilize supplies wisely.
- Maintain productivity standards.
- Prevent industrial accidents.

Step 12: Year-End Evaluation and Environmental Assessment

At the end of the fiscal year, after the financial books are closed, the overall fiscal performance of the institution is evaluated. The actual figures are compared with the environmental assessment that was done for the next year's fiscal budget to determine any significant changes or trends differing from the environmental assessment developed for the coming fiscal year.

Organizations deal differently with changes in environmental assumptions, conditions, and programs. Some institutions revise their figures during the budget year to more closely approximate the actual changes that occur. Other organizations do not actually revise their budgets but rather justify the variances on a monthly basis by explaining the reasons for the variances.

BUDGETING FOR SPECIFIC FINANCIAL RESULTS

In the private sector, organizations develop their operational budgets based on specific profit goals. These goals are called profit margins and are usually set in advance of calculating operational expenses. *Profit margin* is the difference between expenditures and revenues, divided by revenues.

SAMPLE CALCULATIONS

Revenue − expenses = profit ÷ revenue = profit margin
$1,000,000 − $850,000 = $150,000 ÷ $1,000,000 = 15%

In a hospital setting, this methodology is accomplished in the following manner:

1. The CFO, in collaboration with the administrative team, forecasts the next year's units of service and revenues (equivalent to sales forecasts in the private sector).

2. The administrative team reviews objectives and identifies profit goals.

3. The predetermined profit goal is subtracted from the forecasted profit goals. The remaining funds constitute the budget expenditures the organization can utilize to meet the projected revenue goals.

EXAMPLE

Forcasted revenue − profit = budgeted expenditures
$1,000,000 − $150,000 = $850,000
Profit ÷ revenues = profit margin
$150,000 ÷ $1,000,000 = 15%
Forecasted revenue × profit margin = profit
$1,000,000 × 15% = $150,000
Forecasted revenue − profit = Budgeted expenses
$1,000,000 − $150,000 = $850,000

FLEXIBLE OPERATING BUDGETS

Flexible operating budgets change as the volume of the business changes. In a hospital setting, as patient days increase or decrease, expenses flex up or down in a predetermined manner to reflect the variation in volume of the service provided. Fixed costs are not flexible, and therefore budget flexibility is directly tied to the variable costs that result from an increase or decrease in patient days. These variable costs include the salaries of direct care givers, medical supplies, meals, and so on. The fixed overhead costs of management salaries, administration, and operation of plant do not vary with patient volume and so do not change in a flexible budget.

Figure 4-1 displays these fixed and variable costs graphically.[1] This graph displays fixed costs as a constant, irrespective of patient days or the volume of service that is delivered. Variable costs are added to fixed costs, or overhead, to determine the total costs of delivering patient care. In understanding this diagram, an important concept is the break-even point. This is the point at which total costs equal revenue received for patient care. Below the break-even point, the unit operates at a loss, and the unit operates at a profit above the break-even point.

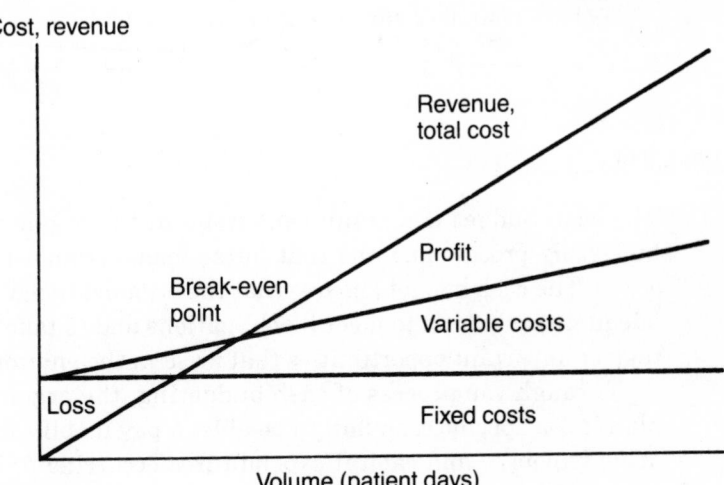

Figure 4-1. *Fixed and variable costs = total costs.*

As patient days or volume decreases, it is important for managers to decrease their variable costs in relation to the decrease in volume. In nursing departments, acuity systems allow nursing managers to decrease their variable costs by staffing only for the actual patients for a particular shift. However, if the census declines below the point of minimum staffing levels, the fixed-cost expenditures will exceed revenues. It is when census or volume drops below minimum staffing patterns (fixed costs) that managers must consider consolidating patients and closing units or assigning patients in a manner that maintains a census on each unit that covers the fixed costs of minimum staffing patterns.

For example, on a medical-surgical unit, minimum staffing is two nurses at all times. If the standard of care on the unit is 5.0 HPPD, census needs to always be maintained at a level of 10.7 patients to cover the fixed costs of the minimum staffing level of two nurses on each of three shifts.

SAMPLE CALCULATIONS

Minimum staffing for 24 hours:

7–3	*3–11*	*11–7*
2 Nurses = 16 hours	2 Nurses = 16 hours	2 Nurses = 16 hours
Head nurse = <u>5.7 hours</u>		
21.7 hours		

21.7 hours + 16 hours + 16 hours = 53.7 hours

53.7 hours ÷ 5 HPPD = 10.7 patients (minimum census)

CASH BUDGET

The cash budget is a significant issue in the organization's budgeting process and one that nurse managers must understand. The cash budget ensures that the organization will have adequate cash flows to meet its obligations and to take advantage of important opportunities that arise in the environment.

Through the process of cash budgeting, the organization plans for a specific cash flow to be able to pay its bills for operating expenses and capital expenditures occurring at specific times.[1] The institution's cash flow position is important to maintain its ability to pay its current liabilities, such as employee salaries and medical suppliers' bills. An institution may have many current assets, but if these are tied up in accounts receivable or inventories, it cannot pay employees and suppliers.

The planning and management of a cash budget is the major responsibility of the CFO. The importance of the cash budget cannot be minimized; serious implications may arise for the health care organization if it is mismanaged or ignored. Table 4-8 shows a sample cash budget with a summary of income and expenses for the year.

The cash budget is important to ensure that the organiza-

Table 4-8 Sample Cash Budget (in 000s)

	Activity	*Balance*
First Quarter		
Cash on hand	$10,000	
Income (1st quarter)	5,000	
	$15,000	
Less:		
Expenses	8,000	
Cash balance (deficit)	$ 7,000	$7,000
Second quarter		
Income (2nd quarter)	$9,000	
Less:		
Expenses	10,000	
Quarter balance		($1,000)
Cash balance		$6,000
Third quarter		
Income (3rd quarter)	$4,000	
Less:		
Expenses	6,000	
Quarter balance		($2,000)
Cash balance		$4,000
Fourth quarter		
Income (4th quarter)	$12,000	
Less:		
Expenses	8,000	
Quarter balance		$4,000
Cash balance		$8,000

Summary of income and expenses

	Income	*Expenses*
First quarter	$5,000	$8,000
Second quarter	$9,000	$10,000
Third quarter	$4,000	$6,000
Fourth quarter	$12,000	$8,000
	$30,000	$32,000

tion has enough cash flowing in to meet the obligations for cash flowing out. Managers must be able to provide the finance department with appropriate information on when expenses need to be paid and when additional cash funds are needed.

A hospital can experience cash flow problems in the following situations:

- It has an increase in bad debts.
- It has an increase in days in receivables.
- It experiences low census periods.
- It must pay for large amounts of nonproductive time (sick time, vacation time, etc.), as well as for high levels of productive time during high census times.
- It has liabilities for outstanding bonds and/or interest payments that were not planned for.

METHODS OF BUDGETING FOR EQUIPMENT

There are three categories of business equipment, each budgeted for in a different manner. The three categories of equipment include nominal value assets, expense items, and capital equipment.

Nominal value assets[13] are items that cost between $100 and $500 and have a useful life of more than 1 year. Nominal value assets are not included in the operational budget or the capital equipment budget but are obtained through the completion of an appropriations request.

Expense items cost less than $100, and are budgeted on the operational budget by means of a line item such as equipment, medical supplies, nonmedical supplies, or miscellaneous.

Capital equipment consists of items that cost more than $500, and have a useful life of more than 1 year. The capital budget is developed separately from the operational budget.

Capital Equipment Budget

The *capital budget* outlines the institution's future investments in plant and equipment. The term *plant* refers to the institution's building and major equipment. There are two basic components of a capital budget: the long-term planning or major acquisitions component and the short-term budgeting component. The long-term major acquisitions component outlines future replacement and/or additional expansion programs for the institution that exceed 1 year in length. The short-term component of the capital budget deals with equipment purchases within an annual budget cycle. Examples include purchases such as a nurse call system, hospital beds, monitoring equipment, medication carts, computers, and so on.

The capital budgeting process for a health care institution has been outlined by Berman and Weeks[9]:

1. *Initial budget meeting:* This initial budget meeting is between the department director and the administrative officer to discuss capital equipment needs for the coming year. Tentative agreements on required equipment should be an outcome of this meeting.

2. *Capital equipment budget form:* The department manager completes the capital equipment budget form that includes the following information:

   - Description request
   - Quantity desired
   - Nature of the request (Is it a replacement, renovation, or addition?)
   - Date or quarter requested for purchase
   - Justification of request (an explanation of why the expenditure should be made and the potential benefits received)
   - Priority ranking

   A sample capital equipment budget request form is exhibited in Table 4-9.

3. *Supporting documentation:* Department directors provide supporting material for each proposed capital expenditure. Such supporting material should include the following:

   - The service provided by the capital item
   - The necessity and/or importance of the service provided
   - The expected utilization of the equipment (*e.g.,* 7 days/week, 24 hours/ day = 100% utilization)
   - The expected life of the capital item
   - Capital costs of equipment, including installation, operating and maintenance costs
   - The estimated savings or profits received from the expenditure

Table 4-9   Sample Capital Equipment Budget Request Form

Department _____

Department manager _____

Date _____

Description of Request	Quantity	Nature	Estimate of Cost	Justification	Priority	Date Required

4. *Review of capital budget requests:* The department manager reviews his capital equipment budget request with his administrator. Following review and agreement, the package is forwarded to the chief financial officer for review and analysis.

5. *Review of entire capital equipment budget:* The chief financial officer reviews the entire capital equipment budget with the administrator or president of the institution for prioritization and analysis.

6. *Presentation of capital budget to finance committee of board of directors:* Finance committee makes the decision on the hospital's capital budget. Approved items are included in the final budget.

It must be stated that the process of budgeting for capital varies significantly from one health care institution to another.

The process outlined here was utilized mainly to show the rationale behind most capital budgeting procedures from a generic perspective. Some institutions have many more steps, whereas some have significantly fewer. It is believed that the nurse manager should understand the basic logic and rationale behind the process. Once understood, it is fairly simple to adapt to varying procedures and forms because the underlying theory and rationale are the same.

BUDGETING BY PRODUCT LINE

As institutions increase their computer capacities and access to data on demographics, diagnoses, and product lines, they will increase their budgeting sophistication. As prospective payment systems become more prominent, budgeting by patient days and procedures will be replaced by per case or product line budgeting. Access to historical data regarding past medical cases is an absolute necessity for developing a budget by product line.

Table 4-10 is a sample product line budget for a coronary care unit. The 2,500 patient days were divided into the five major diagnoses or product lines that were historically treated in the unit. Computerized historical data yielded the average length of stay (LOS) and the number of cases experienced for

Table 4-10   Budgeting by Product Line

Cost center _____   Year _____
Capacity: 10   % Occupancy: 70%
Patient days: 2,500

Product Line:	Average LOS	Number of Cases	Patient Days	HPPD/ Product Line	Total Direct Hours of Care
Myocardial infarction	4	300	1,200	15	18,000
Congestive heart failure	2	50	100	18	1,800
Complex medical	6	100	600	16	9,600
Chest pain	2	200	400	12	4,800
Cardiac arrest	2	100	200	20	4,000
Total hours of direct care required = 38,200					

each product line. The original 2,500 patient days can be recovered by multiplying the number of cases per product line by the average LOS for each product line.

The fifth column on the budget is the standard of nursing care that will be delivered to each kind of patient in hours per patient day (HPPD). In a cost-containment environment, it is important to put nursing resources where they are truly needed for specific patient care rather than providing all patients with an average amount of nursing resources.

The final column of total hours of direct care by product line is determined by multiplying the nursing care standard by the number of patient days projected for each product line.

Total hours of direct care for the coronary care unit can be calculated by adding up the total hours of care required for each product line. This method of budgeting for salary expense of direct care givers by product line or patient condition requires considerably more time and data to complete but gives a more accurate forecast of patient volume and labor expenditures required for particular patient mixes.

SUMMARY

The budget is the financial plan for allocating resources to accomplish annual and ongoing goals for a health care organization. Some of the important concepts of budgeting that were covered in this chapter include the following:

1. The budget is a financial master plan, control mechanism, and tool for evaluating the organization's fiscal performance.

2. In the health care industry, 50% to 70% of annual operational expenses are attributed to employee salaries.

3. *Fixed costs* or overhead do not vary with service volume. Examples of fixed costs include management salaries, employee benefits, nonproductive time, financing costs, and depreciation.

4. The *variance report* is the method of using the budget as a control and evaluation tool. Actual figures are compared with budgeted figures on a monthly and year-to-date basis to identify and implement adjustments that need to be made in managing a department or organization.

5. A *full-time equivalent* (*FTE*) is a unit of time that is equivalent to 40 hours of work per week, 80 hours per pay period, and 2,080 hours per year.

6. *Benefit* or *nonproductive time* is the time an organization pays an employee not to work. Examples include sick time, vacation time, and holiday time. Employee benefit costs include the cost of workmen's compensation and health care coverage for employees. These expenses are a significant portion of the acute care budget, if they are not managed effectively.

7. There are four major budget methodologies that are utilized in organizations in their pure state or in combination with each other: *flat percentage increase method, management by objectives, planning, programming, and budgeting,* and *zero-based budgeting.*

8. The three major functions of the budget process include planning, management of programs, and control of spending.

REFERENCES

1. Lusk E, Lusk J: Financial and Managerial Control: A Health Care Perspective. Rockville, MD, Aspen Publications, 1979
2. Koontz H, O'Donnell C: Essentials of Management, McGraw-Hill, 1978
3. Thompson, Strickland: Strategy and Policy. Business Publications, Inc., 1981
4. Lynden F, Miller E: Public Budgeting: Program Planning and Implementation, 4th ed. Englewood Cliffs, NJ, Prentice-Hall, 1982
5. Drucker P: The Practice of Management. New York, Harper & Row, 1954
6. Odiorne G: Management by Objectives. Belmont, CA, 1965
7. Shillinglaw G, Gordon M, Ronen J: Accounting: A Management Approach, 6th ed. Homewood, IL, Richard D Irwin, 1979
8. McGee R: Fundamentals of Accounting and Finance. Englewood Cliffs, NJ, Prentice-Hall, A Spectrum Book, 1983
9. Berman H, Weeks L: The Financial Management of Hospitals, 5th ed. Ann Arbor, Health Administration Press, 1982
10. Mitchell F, Cloneer A, Coile R: Multi-scenario Forecasting and Health Management in the 1980's. Presented at the Third International Symposium on Forecasting, in Philadelphia, June 6, 1983
11. Managerial Cost Accounting for Hospitals. Chicago, American Hospital Association, 1980
12. Barkholz D: Cost consciousness gives managers a chance to standardize, centralize. Modern Healthcare July 19, 1985
13. Carr RN: The Promotable Woman. Bellmont, CA, Wadsworth, 1982

ADDITIONAL READINGS

1. Dillion R: Zero-Based Budgeting for Health Care Institutions. Rockville, MD, Aspen Publications, 1979
2. Musgrave R, Musgrave P: Public Finance in Theory and Practice. New York, McGraw-Hill, 1984
3. Horngren C: Cost Accounting, 2nd ed. Englewood Cliffs, NJ, Prentice-Hall, 1967

Marketing Skills for Nurse Administrators

MARKETING is a relatively new concept in the health care industry. In the past, it was not perceived necessary for health care institutions to have expertise in business skills such as marketing. However, with the introduction of competition into health care, marketing has become a necessary business tool, rather than a luxury for acute care institutions.

Marketing is in its developemental stages in the health care industry, even though some organizations have been fairly aggressive in their marketing efforts. Most hospital marketing departments acknowledge only one of the four Ps of marketing. Most hospital marketing departments focus on the public relations and promotions functions, giving little time and resources to the concepts of product, place, and price.

Ten years ago, marketing was a department or function that dealt exclusively with a hospital's community relationships. The marketing function in many hospitals has come a long way in ten years. However, it has a long way to go to help the institution meet the challenges of a competitive environment. As more institutions develop their marketing programs, both the institution and the consumer will benefit from a delivery system that is more responsive to the changing health care needs of the marketplace.

This chapter will attempt to provide the nurse manager/administrator with the fundamental principles and practices of marketing. It includes the application of these principles and practices to the health care industry and practice of nursing. The discipline of marketing has a language of its own, and this chapter includes basic marketing terminology with examples applied to the health care setting.

OBJECTIVES

After completing this chapter, the reader will be able to

1. Identify and transfer specific marketing principles to the health care environment.
2. Outline the methodology for analyzing hospital services by product line.
3. Identify three advantages of product line analysis and management techniques.
4. Identify the four basic components of marketing.
5. Define and utilize basic marketing terminology.
6. Identify three major goals of marketing.

7. Classify hospital products based on their profitability and growth potentials.

8. Outline and understand the four Ps of marketing.

9. Identify and understand two major goals of pricing.

10. Outline the product life cycle of any product.

11. Outline the phases that marketing programs experience.

12. Identify and implement two marketing strategies for your own professional advancement.

13. Identify two marketing strategies for advancing nursing services in a community.

DEFINITION OF MARKETING

Peter Drucker is quoted as saying, "Marketing is so basic that it cannot be considered a separate function" from other functions in the organization. "It is the whole business seen from the point of view of its final result, that is, from the customer's point of view.[1]

Philip Kotler defined marketing as "the exchange processes and relationships that occur in the process of attempting to satisfy human wants and needs," in his popular text *Marketing Management,* which is used in many schools of business today.[2]

Marketing is the link between society's needs and wants, and the responses by the marketplace in terms of the goods and services that are then produced. As was thoroughly outlined in Chapter 1, individual and societal needs and wants are never ending and never fulfilled because resources are always limited. This is an economic principle. The process of exchanging resources for goods and services to meet the needs and wants of the individual, as well as society, is called *marketing.*

The marketer's focus is to track never-ending consumer needs and wants, and then to create the products to meet them. A *need* is defined as a state of felt deprivation, arising out of the human condition. An example of a need is food. Food is needed for one to survive as a human being. A *want* is defined as a desire for a specific satisfier for a need. A steak is an example of a want to satisfy the human need for food. There are many ways to satisfy the need for food. Steak is the preferred way, or the want in this particular case. An example of needs and wants in the health care industry follows:

Need: When an individual is ill, he requires or needs health care services.

Want: When a particular patient is ill, he may want a private room.

Intention is the decision to acquire a specific satisfier for a need or want that accepts certain predetermined terms or conditions. An example of an intention is a patient selecting a private room, agreeing to pay an additional fee above what his insurance company covers.

HISTORY OF MARKETING

Peter Drucker believes that marketing, as we know it, was first begun in Tokyo, Japan, by the Mitsui family around 1650. The Mitsui family operated a form of a modern department store and marketed a variety of products to local consumers based on their needs and wants. Marketing first became visible in the United States in the middle of the 19th century in the International Harvester Company. Cyrus H. McCormick (1809-1889) is credited with making the first U.S. contribution to marketing by inventing the following basic tools of modern marketing[2]:

- Market research
- Market analysis
- Pricing policies

It was not, however, until the early 1900s that the term *marketing* appeared in academic settings.

In the past, the health care industry did not believe that it needed to be skilled in promotion, innovation, market positioning, and other marketing strategies to be successful. Acute care institutions felt that they existed to provide care for "sick"people, without any thought of implementing the business strategies traditionally used by the private sector. It was only in the late 1970s and early 1980s that health care organizations added marketing departments to their organizational charts. In the 1980s it is difficult to pick up a professional health care journal that does not contain at least one article on the marketing of traditional, as well as alternative, health care services.

GOALS OF MARKETING

Marketing strives to accomplish various goals. One of its major goals is to maximize the marketplace's consumption of a company's products or services. Therefore, a company's marketing efforts are geared to increasing the amount of its goods and/or services that will be bought or exchanged for money in the marketplace. A *marketplace* is the environment in which actual and potential buyers and sellers of a product exchange their resources. A *market* is the set of all actual and potential buyers of a product. A *product* is defined as goods and services that are capable of satisfying a need or desire. Examples of products include an object, a service, an activity, a place, and an idea.

A second goal of marketing is to maximize consumer satisfaction. This is accomplished by tracking the changing wants and needs of the consumer, and then targeting a company's production of goods and services to meet those needs and wants. In their popular bestseller, *In Search of Excellence,* Peters and Waterman emphasize the fact that "excellent" companies stay "close to the customer."[3] They believe that this important management function is being commonly overlooked or underestimated in many companies today. This fundamental concept of striving to satisfy a customer's needs and anticipating future desires is considered a key for success. The concept of "staying close to the consumer " is the corner stone of the discipline of marketing. Peters and Waterman describe how excellent companies such as Hewlett-Packard and IBM focus on identifying and meeting the needs and wants of their consumers. These companies implement changes in their operations and products based on their consumers' ongoing perceptions and feedback.

A third-level goal of marketing is ultimately to contribute to the quality of life of an individual or society. This goal includes not only enhancing the quality of life, but also taking responsibility for the negative by-products or results of a particular product or service developed or offered by an organization.

For the first two goals of marketing, success is determined by business profits, whereas the success of the third goal is measured by consumer satisfaction and improved quality of life. The third goal of marketing is not the goal most commonly thought of when marketing is discussed. Traditionally, the business sector has been perceived as very "bottom-line" oriented and preoccupied with profits. Somehow it did not "seem right" for a service-oriented organization such as a hospital to be involved with something so "bottom-line" oriented as marketing. When the third goal is acknowledged, however, it becomes very appropriate for a hospital to be involved in marketing. After all, doesn't the third goal describe what hospitals are all about? Health care institutions can easily identify with the goal of contributing to the quality of life.

MARKETING PHILOSOPHIES OF MANAGEMENT

There are various management philosophies regarding the function and importance of marketing in the organization. These different philosophies determine the role that marketing plays in the organization, as well as the goals of marketing for the organization. There are four management orientations for marketing that determine the entire organization's philosophy and mission in the marketplace. These orientations can usually be traced to the individual manager's previous business experience. They include the production orientation, market orientation, sales orientation, and societal marketing orientation.

1. The *production orientation* assumes that consumers will purchase those products that are affordable and available. Management, therefore needs to focus on the efficient production function, so that the organization can offer a product at a reasonable price and in the amount demanded in the marketplace.

2. The *product orientation* assumes that the consumer purchases products that afford them the most quality for the price. In this orientation, management devotes most of its resources to providing a quality product to the marketplace.

3. The *sales orientation* assumes that the consumers do not buy any more than required by their absolute needs, unless they are stimulated by substantial sales efforts. Management's main job is to maintain a strong sales department to stimulate, attract, and hold customers.

4. The *marketing orientation* believes that the major task of the organization is to identify the needs and wants of the

target market and then create products that meet those needs and wants, more efficiently and conveniently than does the competition. Management's main focus is to research the needs and wants of the target market and then to deliver products that satisfy those needs and wants.

The term *consumer sovereignty* originated from the marketing orientation.[4] *Consumer sovereignty* is a principle of economic efficiency that advocates the production of those goods and services that consumers value most highly. In other words, when a marketplace is influenced by consumer sovereignty it gives precedence to producing those goods and services that consumers value or request most often. Consumers with the most wealth and income influence goods and services that are produced more than the consumers with fewer resources.

The *societal marketing orientation* goes one step further than the marketing orientation and advocates that the goal of the organization is to satisfy wants and needs of a specific target market, while providing society with long-term benefits. This management orientation acknowledges that consumer wants do not always coincide with their individual or society's long-term interests. The company goes on to take responsibility for the long-term effects on society, as well as the individual, for the products it produces to satisfy current wants and needs.

These management orientations are important because they can explain why various organizations operate differently from one another. Their beliefs about consumer behavior and their organizational missions change the focus of operations. When health care organizations implement marketing efforts, management will need to agree on one of these orientations to focus their efforts and resources in the same direction. It is possible for different orientations to be used for different health care services or products. For example, when a health care organization is in the business of drug development, it is preferred that it operate from a societal marketing orientation. If this is the case, it would not put a drug on the market that had not been adaquately tested for long-term side effects. If, however, it were operating from a sales orientation, its goal would be to put all its efforts into selling the drug to consumers without thought of potential long-term effects of the drug on society. In the long run, the company would not benefit from this management orientation, because when side effects are discovered, the company would lose its position in the marketplace.

Another real example of the importance of management orientation in marketing efforts can be cited as a result of the Tylenol incidents that occurred in the early 1980s. When there were numerous deaths resulting from tampering with Tylenol capsules, the manufacturer went to great lengths to remove Tylenol from store shelves, to develop "tamper-proof" packaging, and to do additional promotions to communicate its interest in and concern for the long-term well-being of the nation. After a second incident with Tylenol capsules in 1985, the company went on to discontinue its capsules completely and switch to Tylenol "caplets." The manufacturer clearly exhibited a societal marketing approach in the marketplace and with its target market. As a result, Tylenol is well respected in the marketplace today, and survived an unfortunate experience that could have ruined the company.

THE FOUR P's OF MARKETING

Almost everyone has been exposed to the four P's of marketing at one time or another. McCarthy first made popular this simplified marketing classification system.[2] It is defined as follows:

Product

Promotion

Place

Price

The specific variables that describe and elaborate on each of the four P's are included in Table 5-1.

When these marketing variables are combined in various levels and ways, they form the company's marketing mix. *Marketing mix* is the specific combination of marketing variables that a company chooses to influence its target market to purchase its products. For instance a hospital might choose the following combination of the four P's to market its outpatient surgery program or influence its potential patients to use its outpatient surgery department.

SAMPLE MARKETING MIX FOR "SAME-DAY" SURGERY PROGRAM

Price

List price = $500 for minor procedures
Discounts = Medicare deductible waived on weekends
5% discount for Senior Citizens
Credit terms = 5% discount for cash

Promotion

Advertising = Sent out 100,000 direct-mail pieces
Publicity = Local newspaper wrote full-page story on new "same-day" surgery program

Place

Location = Free-standing "same-day" surgery building with free parking
Transportation = Free pick up and delivery available
Channels = Can be referred by private physician, as well as have minor surgery as a "walk-in"

Product

Quality = Competent staff and physicians, but no-frills building to keep costs reasonable
Packaging = Billed as fast, safe, convenient alternative to inpatient surgery
Options = All minor procedures available under general or local anesthesia
Features = Convenient, reasonable health care service

Table 5-1   Specific Variables of the Four P's

Product	Quality
	Styles
	Various options
	Brand name
	Size
	Packaging
	Color
	Warranty
Place	Channels of distribution
	Coverage
	Method of distribution
	Inventory
	Transportation methods
Promotion	Advertising
	Sales promotions
	Publicity
Price	List price
	Discounts
	Allowances
	Payment period
	Credit terms

This specfic combination of marketing variables has determined a marketing strategy that the hospital feels will influence its target market of outpatient surgery customers to purchase more outpatient surgery services. Each of these variables has been identified because of its perceived ability to meet the needs and desires of the target market for outpatient services. A marketing strategy does not, for example, limit itself to providing a quality product. Each of these variables supposedly contributes to the consumer's perception of the value of the service provided by the program. When the volume of outpatient surgeries is not meeting the goals of the organization, the marketing mix and strategy are re-evaluated. The *marketing strategy* includes the organization's goals and objectives for the product and outlines a plan of action by identifying a marketing mix and the specific allocation of resources to attain those goals. The plan is constantly evaluated and revised based on changes in the environment and increased competition.

Product

As defined earlier, a *product* is a good or service that is capable of satisfying a need or desire. A product can be an object, a service, an activity, a place, or an idea. Table 5-2 shows examples of each of these kinds of products that have traditionally been offered in the health care marketplace.

The concept of product is especially important for health care professionals. In the past, the health care industry identified its products as displayed in Table 5-2. A hospital's products include nursing care, ancillary services, medications, education, and so on. The hospital billed for services based on the number and kind of services that were rendered to the patient.

In the current prospective reimbursement system of Medi-

Table 5-2 Traditional Health Care Products

Kind	Example
Object	Medication
Service	Nursing care
Activity	Physical therapy
Place	Inpatient private rooms
Idea	Stop-smoking program

care DRGs, hospital products have changed to "recovered" patients by diagnosis. The hospital is reimbursed by Medicare and some third-party payors by "recovered " patients, not by the number of medications, services, or ancillary treatments that the patient receives. This is a key marketing concept for hospitals in the 1980s. Hospitals will need to redefine their products to reflect their reimbursement.

Hospital services are classified by various methods because of the specific methods of reimbursement involved. In the case of reimbursement by case, diagnosis, or DRG, the product is a "recovered" patient. The hospital is reimbursed by the number of "recovered " patients by diagnosis upon discharge rather than by the number of tests, medications, or treatments it provides to these inpatients.

In the case of third-party payors contracting for per diem rates, the product remains patient days. In per diem or per day contracting, third-party payors negotiate flat per day rates with hospitals to care for any of their patients admitted to the institutions. The rate is usually determined irrespective of the diagnosis of the patient. (Please refer to Chapter 1 for the economic implications of per diem reimbursement.)

At the present time, emergency services, home health visits, outpatient services, and ambulatory surgery services are still reimbursed on a cost basis, with various "caps" or ceiling payments. There is a good chance, however, that these services will also be reimbursed by alternative prospective methods in the future.

PRODUCT LINE ANALYSIS AND MANAGEMENT

The changing concept of "product " in health care has led to many articles and discussions about the application of product line analysis and management in the acute care setting.[5] *Product line analysis* is a method of analyzing products in terms of inputs and outputs. This analysis categorizes the services or products that a hospital provides into product lines. A *product line* is composed of similar services that are grouped together to manage costs, process, quality, and marketing of the service more efficiently. The historic unit of service in the hospital has been a patient day and/or specific procedures. Because of Medicare per case reimbursement, patient day is not the only unit of service that administration should focus on in the management of the institution.

If and when an institution makes the decision to reorganize its operations by product line, there are some factors to consider before making these changes.

1. Product lines should be defined as broadly as possible. An institution does not want to deal with an unmanageable number of product lines.
2. Product lines should be medically meaningful to gain physician and professional support.
3. Resource use per case should be relatively homogenous across a product line.
4. The data used to establish a product line must have statistical validity.

Product line analysis and management is the defining and analyzing of hospital products and services in terms of total resource use per case and the making of management decisions based on that analysis. Product line analysis is built on total cost accounting principles (see Chapter 3). The determination of actual cost per case is critical. All hospital costs for an admission are tracked by diagnosis, physician, and payor. In addition, all hospital fixed overhead costs are allocated to actual patients or product lines. In product line analysis, all costs from admission to discharge are calculated and compared with the reimbursement per case. Even though patient days has less significance than in the past, it is important to track length of stay by product line or diagnosis. It may be that daily costs for inpatient care are reasonable, but the patient's length of stay is too long, causing the total cost per case to be greater than the reimbursement per case.

Other terms that have appeared in the current business and health care literature related to product line include *strategic business unit (SBU)* and *strategic program unit (SPU).*[6] An SBU is defined as a group of products that is offered to a clearly defined market and requires its own specific marketing strategy. An SPU describes a program or service that is offered to a specialized market. The term was identified especially for the health care industry to describe the unique patient care aspects of health products. Both SBUs and SPUs include the financial aspect of the unit from a cost and reimbursement perspective.

Tracking Costs in Product Line Analysis. Figure 5-1 is a simple form that outlines a methodology for analyzing costs by product line. On the horizontal axis, the product lines are identified. The vertical axis enumerates various services that the institution provides. Above the double line are routine services or various levels of nursing services. Most acute care institutions provide three basic levels of inpatient nursing care: critical care nursing, intermediate nursing care, and medical-surgical nursing. These services are referred to as routine services because all inpatients require a nurse, room, and board. Specific services appearing below the double line are not provided to all patients or in the same quantities. Patients receive services in various combinations and intensities based on their diagnosis and physician practice patterns.

By obtaining computerized data from the medical records or billing departments, it is possible to fill in the number of days a particular type of patient spent on a medical floor, critical care unit, and so on, from admission to discharge. It is possible to multiply the length of stay in each level of care by the average cost per day in those units. (Cost per unit of service is calculated in Chapter 3.)

The next step is to identify the number of x-rays, CT scans, ultrasounds, and laboratory tests the patient had during his entire hospital stay. (The list of treatments in Figure 5-1 is not all inclusive.) The number of each type of procedure or treatment is then multiplied by the cost per unit of service for each procedure. (The total cost per unit of service for each of these procedures is calculated by utilizing full cost-accounting techniques discussed in detail in Chapter 3.)

Table 5-3 shows how this product line cost data is compared with the reimbursement per DRG. For example, DRG 122, or acute myocardial infarction, routinely averages 4.5 days of medical-surgical nursing care at the routine cost per day of $146. DRG 122 historically requires 4 days of critical care service at the routine cost of $516 per day. Radiology treatments cost $412, (calculated by multiplying the number of radiology treatments by the average cost per unit of service for radiology), laboratory costs are $545, respiratory therapy treatments are $460, pharmacy costs are $355, and miscellaneous or other services cost $718 per case. This $5,184, if properly calculated,

	Cardiovascular	Orthopedics	Cardiology	General surgery	Ophthalmology
Patient data					

Patient days/cost

	Cardiovascular	Orthopedics	Cardiology	General surgery	Ophthalmology
Medical nursing					
Surgical nursing					
Critical care nursing					
Operating room					
Obstetrical nursing					
Pediatric nursing					

Treatments/cost

	Cardiovascular	Orthopedics	Cardiology	General surgery	Ophthalmology
DX radiology					
X-ray					
CT scan					
Ultrasound					
Respiratory					
Treatments					
Respirator					
EEG					
EKG					
EMG					
Physical therapy					
Laboratory					
Operating room time					

Figure 5-1.   *Product line information.*

represents the total hospital costs for a cardiology patient at this institution and accounts for this patient's portion of total hospital costs.

Proceeding down to the bottom of Table 5-3, revenue per DRG or the Medicare payment to the institution for this acute myocardial infarction is compared with the total cost to care for the patient. This revenue figure of $5,349 is payment in full for the care of acute MI patients at this institution. The institution receives no other funds from Medicare for this patient's care. By utilizing product line analysis, it is possible to see that DRG 122 yields a net profit of $165 per case. It is possible to see where all the institution's costs are located to deliver care to this patient. If the cost exceeds the reimbursement, it is easy to identify where excessive expenses are located to make the appropriate reductions.

Using product line analysis, it is possible to look at length of stay in each product line by nursing level of care, to determine if reductions are needed and possible. Utilizing product line analysis, reductions that need to be made in areas other than nursing can be identified. Ancillary cost per case is calculated and then the appropriate reductions can be made by answering these kinds of questions:

- Do all patients need daily laboratory work?
- Is it really beneficial to wake patients up around the clock for every 4-hour respiratory treatment?

Table 5-3   Product Line Analysis

| DRG# | Nursing Services | | Ancillary Services | | | | | |
	Med–Surg	Spec Care	Rad	Lab	Resp	Pharm	Other	Total
122	4.5 days $630	4 days $2064	$412	$545	$460 ⁴	$355	$718	$5184
107	12 days $1752	4 days $2064	$600	$950	$1200	$1600	$14,431	$22,597
127	6 days $876	3 days $1548	$350	$300	$250	$300	$250	$3,874

DRG#	Revenue/DRG	Cost/DRG	Net Profit/Loss
122	$5,349	$5,184	$165
107	$15,000	$22,597	−$7,597
.127	$4,174	$3,874	$300

- Are our interventions really beneficial to the patient in the volume and frequency they are performed?

Product Line Management by Medical Committee. Management of patient care by product line or by diagnosis requires a great deal of cooperation and collaboration among physicians, hospital administraton, and professional staff. The medical committee structure seems a likely place to organize and accomplish this task. The medical committee to manage a specific product line of patient care should include physicians, administration, and professional staff. The committee should review cost and reimbursement data by diagnosis and physician for the purpose of determining goals for length of stay and desired treatment modalities necessary to target the cost of treatment per diagnosis below the reimbursement per case. Physicians and nurses need to collaborate on the medical and nursing interventions desired to accomplish this goal. Administration will focus on implementing or changing policies and procedures that facilitate the efficiency of this collaborative effort. Motivation to accomplish these goals stems from the common desire to have the institution survive, so that physicians and professional staff have a place to practice, and so that the community can maintain its access to health care services. The following is an outline of the advantages and disadvantages of product line analysis and management as tools to be implemented in the health care institution.

ADVANTAGES AND DISADVANTAGES OF PRODUCT LINE ANALYSIS

Advantages

Shows relationship of inputs to outputs
Gives profit and loss information for a line or service
Attaches all costs to a specific service
Provides better control and review of total resources
Increases everyone's cost awareness
Promotes more detailed planning
Increases team work among hospital departments
Promotes increasing efficiency within a product line
Promotes better decision making

Disadvantages

New management tool requiring education in health field
Resistance due to the newness of tool
Requires computerized services

INTERMEDIATE PRODUCTS

Currently, in the case of Medicare's DRG reimbursement and per diem contracting, there is a class of products called *intermediate products*. Examples of these intermediate products include ancillary services such as laboratory tests, respiratory therapy treatments, radiology treatments, EKGs, and CT scans. These intermediate services contribute to producing the inpatient "product" of a recovered patient but are not specifically reimbursed for by the number of the services that are delivered.

A laboratory test is considered a product or service as an outpatient procedure, and is reimbursed by specific test. That same laboratory test in the inpatient setting is termed an intermediate service and is not specifically reimbursed for by each test. A hospital might therefore decide to increase its promotion of outpatient laboratory services, yet attempt to minimize laboratory procedures that physicians order for inpatients.

Other classifications of hospital products or services include general services and specialty services. *General services* are the routine inpatient services that a hospital provides, whereas *speciality products* are defined as highly differentiated services that require specific technology and training. An example of a specialty product in a hospital would be an open heart surgery program.

Hospitals are being forced to make decisions on which products it has the expertise to provide, as well as which products or services it can afford to provide, based on its case mix, product line analysis, and future goals. If the reimbursement for a specialty service, such as open heart surgery, is very low, it may be very difficult for the hospital to maintain costs below reimbursement for that product. If the institution cannot make up the losses on other products, they may need to "dump" the program, so that the institution can survive.

BOSTON CONSULTING GROUPS PRODUCT CLASSIFICATION SYSTEM

In 1979 the Boston Consulting Group developed a classification system for products to identify marketing strategies for various products.[7] The classification system is based on the product's potential growth possibilities and potential profitability. Figure 5-2 shows the product classification matrix.

- Products that have low growth potential but are currently highly profitable are called *cash cows*. The marketing strategy is to maintain them and use the profits to finance other ventures and offset other losses.

- Products that have high growth potential and are currently profitable are called *rising stars*. The market strategy for rising stars is to invest promotional money and management time in them to increase the volume of sales. After a period of increasing growth, rising stars usually become cash cows.

- Products that have high growth potential but are not currently very profitable are called *question marks*. The marketing strategy for question marks can be tricky and risky. One strategy is to attempt to increase volume by aggressive marketing and thereby increase profitability.

- Products that have low growth and profitability potential are called *dogs*. Organizations usually benefit by divesting themselves of dogs because they only place a drain on the organization.

This matrix system is a helpful tool for managers to classify their particular products for the purpose of making intelligent marketing decisions.

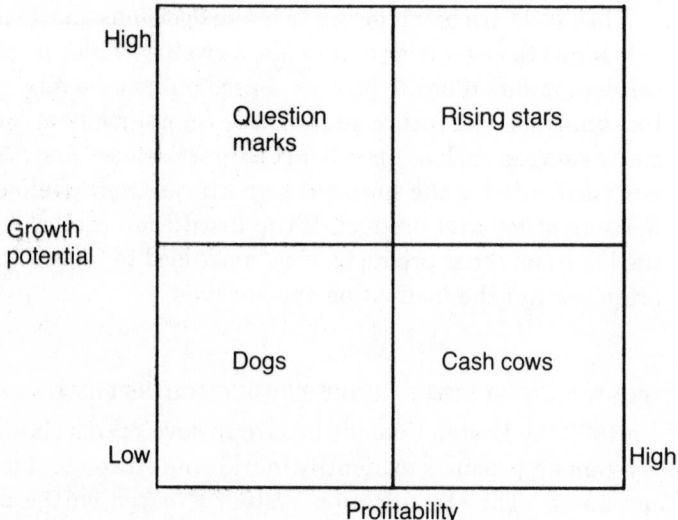

Figure 5-2. *Boston Consulting Group's product matrix.*

EXAMPLE

A medical–surgical head nurse is experiencing a declining census on her floor, and the nurses are being called off on a daily basis. She wants to identify a plan for increasing census so that there is more work available and more revenue for the institution. She could implement the following steps:

1. Identify the "products" delivered on the unit.

2. Classify each product based on the Boston Consulting Group's matrix.

3. Identify a marketing plan to increase the volume of the stars, cash cows, and possibly the question marks on the floor.

PRODUCT LIFE CYCLE

There are typically four stages that a product passes through after its initial creation. These four stages are called the *product life cycle*[8]:

1. The *introduction stage* is the beginning stage of a new product. The organization is usually unsure of the product's growth potential and the consumer's response to or demand for the product.

2. The *growth stage* occurs when innovators enter the market, and expand its total size. Marketing strategies are geared to increasing the size of the market or number of consumers for the product.

3. The *maturity stage* begins when competition enters the market to obtain a share of the market. The market for the product is at its peak in the maturity stage. Marketing strategies for a product in this stage are aimed at increasing the organization's share of the market. This can be accomplished by converting consumers of other products to users of your products. Inpatient care has been identified in this stage in the 1980s.

4. The *market decline stage* is the stage when the size of the market decreases because of new technology, new ideas or products, or changes in consumer needs. In this stage, the advertising budget is greatly reduced in favor of the company's other products.

There are some definite similarities between the Boston Consulting Group's Classification System and the product life cycle of most products. Table 5-4 compares the two models and describes their similarities.

As health care organizations attempt to meet the challenges of increasing competition, product diversification and vertical integration become increasingly popular marketing strategies.

Table 5-4   Comparing Two Marketing Models

Boston Consulting Group's Martrix	Product Life Cycle	Similar Characteristics
1. Question marks	Introductory stage	Future risky High growth potential
2. Rising stars	Growth stage	High growth potential High profitability
3. Cash cows	Maturity stage	High profitability Low growth potential
4. Dogs	Decline stage	Decreasing growth Decreasing profitability

Product diversification is the concept of expanding products and product lines into new areas. In the past, hospitals concentrated on treating sick people. As they adopt an attitude of product diversification, they expand into day-care surgery, home health, and wellness programs. *Vertical integration* is the concept of adding products to an organization that increases their control of more functions. An example is when a hospital develops a home health agency of its own and no longer refers its patients to an outside agency, thereby gaining more control over its patient population and flow.

SUMMARY

The first step an organization takes in developing a market plan is to identify the products it currently delivers based on its reimbursement. Is reimbursement determined by "recovered" patients, patient days, general services, specialty services, or all of the above? The institution then identifies the cost of producing the various products it supplies to the marketplace, utilizing full cost-accounting techniques. The cost to deliver the services is compared with the reimbursement of that service to identify the "winners and losers."

Loser products are analyzed for production efficiency, and potential cost reductions are implemented. After making all possible reductions without adversely affecting the quality of the product, management makes appropriate decisions on whether to continue to provide the service.

Promotion

Promotion is the marketing function that communicates information about the product to the marketplace. Marketing is often defined solely in terms of the promotion function or advertising. It is important to note that the success or failure of a particular marketing effort is first determined by identifying the right product. A good promotional campaign for a poor product ultimately results in failure. A good marketing plan consists of the appropriate combination of the four P's, with product always coming first.

The goal of the promotion or communication function in marketing is to move the consumer from a position of ignorance about a product to purchase of the product. A simplified model of this desired movement is represented in Figure 5-3.

Marketing tools in the promotion or communication of specific products are called "promotools"[8]. Promotools include publicity programs, point-of-purchase displays, catalogs, films, special packaging, advertising, etc. The four major classifications are the following:

1. *Advertising* is any paid form of promotion of ideas, programs, goods, or services.
2. *Personal selling* is an oral presentation by a seller to a potential buyer for the purpose of selling a product.
3. *Sales promotions* are short-term incentives to encourage the purchase of a product.
4. *Publicity* is a promotion that is not paid for by the company.

According to the model, promotional tools strive to

- Attract the attention of the consumer.
- Stimulate consumer interest in the product.
- Create a desire for the product in the mind of the consumer.

Company action ⟶ Response by marketplace

Promotional effort ⟶ Attention ⟶ Interest ⟶ Desire ⟶ Action

Figure 5-3. *Effect of promotion in marketing.*

- Motivate the consumer into the action of purchasing the product.

An institution or company must guard against implementing a promotional program that deceives or discriminates in the marketplace. Printed promotional materials are more subject to criticism because they can be used as concrete evidence. Hospitals and health care professionals must be particularly careful not to deceive or descriminate in their advertising efforts because the public expects them to be above such questionable activities. The public expects to be able to trust health care providers. Once that trust is betrayed, a health care institution could actually lose a lot more than it ever hoped to gain fron a promotion.

Specific kinds of advertising that health care providers should avoid include the following:

- False and/or misleading advertising. False advertising is self explanatory, whereas misleading advertising is a distortion of information in advertising. The Federal Trade Commission has the capability of issuing a temporary restraining order against advertising that is misleading.
- Bait advertising. Bait advertising attracts buyers with an exceptionally good buy, and then tries to substitute an inferior product.

PROMOTIONAL TOOLS

There are many promotional tools within each one of the classifications already mentioned that can be used in marketing specific products and services. The effectiveness of or the results obtained by the various tools or strategies depends on the resources available for the promotional campaign.

After identifying the right product, the appropriate promotional strategies for the specific product are chosen. Examples of promotional tools include the following:

1. Word of mouth referrals. Many marketers believe this is one of the most effective marketing strategies. They believe that a satisfied customer is the best testimony for the product. On the other hand, word of mouth can also become the most distorted form of promotion. If you have ever played the game "telephone," in which one person whispers a statement to another, with the process continuing through a number of additional people, you know how the original statement can become distorted. This same

phenomenon can occur with word of mouth advertising and could prove to have serious negative effects for the organization.

2. Newspaper articles. Local newspapers are always in need of community service articles. Such articles are essentially free advertising for an organization. It is important for health care managers of various programs or services to maintain a good rapport with the press, to be able to take advantage of this promotional strategy. Nursing administrators and managers need to get out into the community and establish relationships with the press, as well as with other community organizations. Nursing leaders have not done this in the past, and all managers may not be comfortable in this public relations role. The nurse manager can obtain greater access to newspaper coverage, as well as word of mouth referrals, by actively being involved in some manner with the PTA, Chamber of Commerce, and auxillaries in the community. This is a new role for the nurse manager but one that can prove to be very beneficial to the institution and the overall image of the nursing department. It can also prove to be very rewarding for the nurse administrator/manager.

3. Public service announcements. All radio and television stations have an obligation designated by the Federal Communications Commission (FCC) to broadcast a certain number of community or public service announcements. This is another free promotional strategy. These public service announcements can promote services such as health fairs, blood pressure screening programs, and so on. These services draw the consumer to the institution for a promotional activity. The supposition is that when the consumer requires other health care services, he has already established a tie with the facility, and will go to that facility to satisfy future health care needs.

4. Printed materials. Examples of effective promotional printed materials include items that are referred to on an ongoing basis, such as calendars, telephone stickers, matches, and pens. In the health care field, additional examples could include first-aid booklets, poison control booklets, diet information, exercise booklets, and so on. These items have educational benefit, as well as advertising the institution in the marketplace.

5. Paid advertising. It is becoming increasingly popular for hospitals and physicians to pay for advertising in newspapers, magazines, telephone directories, radio, and television. Trevor Fisk,[9] Vice President for Marketing and Plan-

ning at Cooper Hospital/University Medical Center, Camden, NJ, outlines five basic suggestions for hospitals in designing their printed layouts for paid advertising in magazines and newspapers:

- Arouse the reader's interest in the product or service—don't assume it. An example is to offer a free gift such as a health information class.

- Illustrate the product, not the process. For example, for a health care layout, include a picture of a healthy person, such as a runner, rather than a picture of the hospital building. The picture should represent someone with whom the market audience wants to identify.

- Place the organization's name in the headline. Few people read an entire ad. The ad should tell the reader at a glance that he can obtain services to make him look healthy, like the person in the picture, at the place in the headline.

- List the benefits to the individual in the ad. People want to know, "What's in it for me?"

- Include a method to obtain immediate feedback on the advertising. An example for a newspaper or magazine ad is a coupon that can be clipped and mailed in or brought in personally. This allows tracking of the number of customers using the services as a result of the advertising efforts.

6. Introductory offers. In the private sector, introductory offers have been a very effective advertising strategy. Examples include free samples and two-for-one sales. Hospitals have not used this strategy extensively in the past. Examples of introductory offers in the health care setting include free lectures on alcohol and drug dependency for family members of chemically dependent persons, free blood pressure screenings, and so on.

7. Sales calls. Sales calls are a method of communication whereby the organization sends out a representative to another organization to discuss the products and services they could provide the second company. In the health care industry, it has become common for representatives of alcohol and drug programs, occupational or industrial medicine programs, and wellness programs to make sales calls on businesses to inform them of these services that are available to their employees. In the future, it will be more commonplace for nursing administrators and managers to make sales calls to businesses for their home

health, ambulatory care, and educational programs. This might take the form of *field selling* or *executive selling.* Field selling is the act of approaching a company to inform it of the specific services offered by the acute care institution. Executive selling is used when the nurse executive takes a company executive to lunch to sign a contract for a wellness program for the company's employees.

The seven promotional tools outlined here are not all inclusive. Table 5-5 contains a more detailed listing of examples of the specific promotional tools by broad classification.

Management decisions regarding the specific promotional or communicational tool to use for a product depend on the answers to the following questions:

1. What are the goals or objectives of the promotional campaign?

2. What are the company's available resources for promotion of the product?

3. How should the promotional budget be divided among the various promotional tools?

Table 5-5 Promotional Tools

Major Classification of Tool	Example
1. Advertising	Printed materials such as calendars, newsletters, booklets, matches, etc.
	Direct mail
	Fliers
	Billboard advertising
	Ads in newspapers, magazines, and journals
2. Personal selling	Executive selling
	Sales calls
	Fund raising
	Lobbying
3. Sales promotions	Coupons
	Discounts
	Free samples
	Incentives
	Free lectures
	Med-card credit cards
	Introductory offers
4. Publicity	Public service announcements
	Word of mouth
	Interviews
	Blood pressure screenings
	Health fairs
	Speakers bureau
	Public relations

4. What is the target market's perceptions of the product?
5. What stage of the product life cycle is the product currently in?

   Allocation of specific resources for each promotional tool is based on the answers to these questions, as well as the amount of resources available.

PHYSICIAN PROMOTIONS

A final consideration regarding promotional activities for hospitals includes the concept of physicians as distributors or intermediate customers of the acute care institution. If an institution values the physician's role in the delivery of health care services, it will not spend all its marketing dollars on the end consumer, or the patient. The distributor or physician can still influence to some exent, where a patient is admitted for inpatient services and, therefore, warrants attention in the marketing campaign. Marketing efforts aimed at the physician include free meals, parking facilities, physician lounges, dinner parties, and recognition, as well as other amenities.

The marketing efforts targeted at the physician community have created extensive resentment in the nursing community during recent years. However, it is time that the profession of nursing face the facts, and acknowledge that physicians do have a great influence and impact on bringing the consumer into the acute care institution. Like it or not, in the inpatient health care setting, nursing depends on the medical profession for its clients.

Pricing

Pricing is the element of the marketing mix that generates revenue for the organization. All organizations, for-profit and not-for-profit, need to identify specific prices for their products. Pricing is considered by modern marketers as the second most important factor, after product in the marketing mix. Price determinations depend on the factors of cost of the product, demand for the product, and competition.

The concept of price is known by various names, including fee, charge, tuition, rent, and fare. *Pricing strategy* is defined as the range of prices and changes in prices over time, that can accomplish the profit goals and market positioning of the company for a product. *Price making* is the task of setting specific prices when a situation of perfect market competition does not exist. This procedure can be very difficult and complex in the absence of competition because competition creates some guidelines for price setting. *Pricing objectives* are goals for specific profits, revenues, and market share for a product. Because demand for a product depends on the price, each different price for a product results in varying levels of profit, revenue, and market share for the product. The critical aspect is identifying the price that will accomplish the company's goals for profit, revenue, and market share.

There are six major goals that various pricing strategies seek to attain. These major pricing goals are outlined in Table 5-6.

As identified earlier, there are essential factors important in setting prices, regardless of the company's specific goals and objectives. These factors include the cost of the product, the demand for the product, and the competition. There are pricing strategies that acknowledge these various factors. Companies use these various strategies based on their perception of which factors have the greatest impact or implication for their products in the marketplace. Table 5-7 outlines these three impor-

---

Table 5-6 Major Pricing Goals

Pricing Goals/Objectives	*Explanation*
1. Profit-maximizing pricing	Strives to determine the maximum price that the demand for a product will bear.
2. Market-share pricing	Strives to identify the price that maximizes a company's share of the market. Short-term profits are sacrificed for long-term market domination. Profits are believed to follow the market domination.
3. Market-skimming pricing	Includes a high price with a high profit, based on the assumption that the product is in high demand or has no competition.
4. Promotional, loss-leader, and prestige pricing	Sets the price significantly higher or lower than the cost of the product, to accomplish its purpose. Loss-leader pricing is setting the price lower than the cost or the competition to introduce the consumer to the company's products. The company makes up its losses when the consumer purchases other products. An example is a one-cent sale. Prestige pricing is setting unusually high prices to convey the image of a quality product through the pricing function.
5. Target-profit pricing	To attain a satisfactory profit.
6. Current-revenue pricing	To maximize current revenue for the company.

Table 5-7   Pricing Factors and Methods

Pricing Factor	Pricing Method	Definition
Cost of product	1. Mark-up pricing	Determined by multiplying cost by a certain percentage.
	2. Cost-plus pricing	Determined by adding a fixed amount to the cost.
	3. Target pricing	Price is the one that yields a specific profit above the total costs at a particular demand level.
Demand for product	1. Perceived-value pricing	The price is based on the consumer's perceptions of the value of the product.
	2. Price-discrimination pricing	The price of a product varies from one consumer to another, one time to another, and one place vs. another, based on the perceptions of value. Example: seasonal hotel rates.
Competition	1. Going-rate pricing	Determined by the collective wisdom of the marketplace, and is the price the market will bear.
	2. Sealed-bid pricing	This pricing is the lowest price a company is willing to be paid for a product, given that other competitors are vying for the contract.

tant pricing factors and specific pricing strategies that acknowledge the important role of each factor.

PRICING IN HEALTH CARE

Pricing is the marketplace function that hospitals have significantly overlooked in the past. Under a retrospective reimbursement system, maximum net revenues were obtained by averaging total costs and then identifying prices based on that average cost. In the current prospective reimbursement environment, there are other variables that need to be acknowledged in the pricing of hospital services. The Medicare DRG reimbursement figures or prices are based on averaging the cost of care actually delivered by diagnosis. If hospital costs exceed that average cost, the hospital loses money. If hospital costs are less than the average price, the hospital makes money.

Third-party payors also have recently discovered that they can significantly influence the price they pay for health care services by a process called contracting. *Contracting* is a process of competitive bidding between a third-party payor and one or more acute care institutions. Contracting has changed the focus of pricing in health care from cost-based to market-based.

Sealed-bid pricing (Table 5-7) is the pricing method that describes the contracting method of pricing

Place or Distribution

The final P is place or the distribution function of getting the product to the consumer. The distribution of products includes these factors:

1. Channels of distribution
2. Locations of distribution
3. Inventory
4. Transportation of products

The *marketing channel* is the set of institutions that perform the necessory function of moving a product from production to consumption. In other words, all the processes and functions that intervene between a product's production and the consumer's purchase of the product are called marketing channels.

EXAMPLE

The marketing channels for fresh fruit could include the following:
- Channel 1 — Farm worker that picks fruit
- Channel 2 — Trucking company that ships the fruit to the store
- Channel 3 — Grocery store that sells the fruit

Each of the channels in the example is called a channel level. A *direct-marketing channel* consists of no actual channels. An example of a direct-marketing channel is when the product is sold directly to the consumer by the producer. When a farmer invites the public to pick their own apples at $1 a bushel, he has no actual market channel to the consumer. In this example, there are no "middle men" between the producer of the product (the farmer) and the consumer of the product (the apple-picker).

When products travel through various channels from the producer to the buyer, the channels are called *intermediary channels*. One-level channels have one intermediary channel. A retail market is an example of a one-channel market. The retailer is between the producer of the product and the consumer of the product (Fig. 5-4).

A two-level channel has two intermediaries. In the market-place, the most common example consists of the wholesaler and

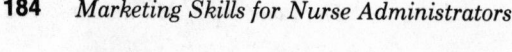

Producer ⟶ Retailer ⟶ Consumer

Drug company ⟶ Hospital ⟶ Patient

Figure 5-4. *Example of a one-level intermediary channel.*

the retailer channels that function between the producer and the consumer (Fig. 5-5).

Health care delivery systems are examples of marketing channels to distribute health care services. Within a health care system, various products are moved from the producer to the consumer by way of various channel levels. Producers of products use particular channels for various reasons. Two of those reasons are as follows:

1. It is fairly costly to market products directly to the consumer. It takes less capital to distribute products through intermediaries, and therefore, capital can be retained to use for other company goals such as growth and development of technology.

2. The intermediaries usually have more expertise in distribution and can be more efficient for that function than the producer.

Producers constantly strive to identify the most effective and efficient number and kind of channels to distribute their products to the consumer. An organization can have a quality product, a competitive price, and an excellent promotional campaign, yet have serious problems because of inefficient marketing channels, too many channels, or the wrong channels. To avoid some of these problems, there are some major functions or tasks of marketing channels that assist the decision maker in identifying the appropriate channels to use. Appropriate marketing channels provide these functions:

1. Research—the gathering of appropriate information and data to plan the exchange function for a particular product.

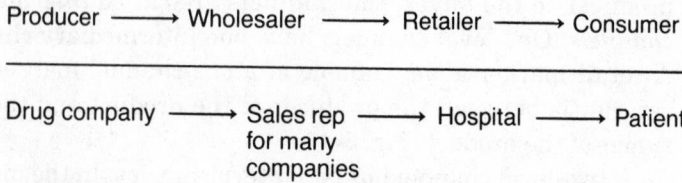

Producer ⟶ Wholesaler ⟶ Retailer ⟶ Consumer

Drug company ⟶ Sales rep for many companies ⟶ Hospital ⟶ Patient

Figure 5-5. *Example of a two-level intermediary channel.*

2. Promotion—the communication of information about the exchange process.

3. Contact—seeking out and communicating with potential buyers.

4. Matching—the designing of the final product to the buyer's specifications; includes activities such as packaging and assembling.

5. Negotiation—the process of agreement on a price and other options to move the product from the producer to the consumer.

6. Physical distribution—the physical transportation, storing, and/or inventorying of the goods.

7. Financing—the identification and distribution of funds to cover the cost of the channels.

8. Risk-taking—the assumption by the intermediary channels of a measure of financial risk in moving goods from the producer to the consumer. The producer actually uses intermediaries for the purpose of decreasing his risk.

Channel intermediaries are called various names in the marketplace. A few of the kinds of channel intermediaries are defined below:

Agent: An agent is a person or company that represents a producer in selling his products, but does not take possession of the products. An example of an agent in the health care industry is a drug manufacturer's representative, who sells drugs to a hospital but does not actually work for the drug company. These kinds of agents represent many drug companies with different product lines.

Broker: A broker is an agent who represents either the seller or the buyer to negotiate a sale or exchange.

Dealer: A dealer buys and resells merchandise either as a retailer or a wholesaler.

Retailer: A retailer buys merchandise and sells it directly to the ultimate consumer.

Wholesaler: A wholesaler buys and resells merchandise to retailers and other buyers. A wholesaler rarely sells to the ultimate consumer.

DIRECT MARKETING SYSTEMS

Direct marketing, or zero-level channel marketing, has become increasingly popular in the 1980s. Examples of various types of direct marketing include the following:

1. Mail-order selling: In mail-order selling, the consumer purchases a product directly from the producer by ordering from a catalog. This is accomplished by mail or a telephone order. There is no middle-man in direct selling.

2. Mass-media selling: In the past few years, producers of records and small appliances have placed ads in newspapers and on television and radio instructing the consumer to contact the producer of the product directly by telephone or mail to receive a product.

3. Door-to-door selling: Door-to-door selling is an example of direct marketing by on-premise selling. The Fuller Brush Company and Avon are two of the most well-known companies that have implemented on-premise selling very successfully.

MARKET RESEARCH

Market research is defined as the collection, organization, analysis, and interpretation of internal and external marketing data for an organization. Analysis of the internal environment yields information about the strengths and weaknesses of the organization, whereas analysis of the external environment provides clues to the opportunities and threats in the marketplace for the organization. A good marketing plan includes knowledge and in-depth analysis of all these factors. A marketing plan that does not acknowledge or fully understand the presence and impact of these factors has been developed in a vacuum and has little insight to assist the organization in meeting its specific goals.

Marketing data can be quantitative or qualitative in nature. Quantitative data is obtained from surveys and questionnaires, and the results obtained from the sample are generalized for the marketplace. Qualitative data is obtained through direct interviews and is used when the marketer is seeking to understand the whys of specific consumer behavior and/or perceptions of value. It is less appropriate to use data from interviews than data from surveys in making generalizations for larger group behavior.

The data and implications gained from polling consumers is invaluable in the rapidly changing health care environment. In the past, health care institutions focused on providing the highest quality of care and service available. Cost was never considered an issue. Arthur Sturm, of Communications Group, Inc., quotes figures indicating that as high as 43% of health care consumers participate in deciding which health care facility they use.[10] Professional Research Consultants, Inc., of Omaha, Nebraska, believes that the percentage is as high as 61%.[11] In either case, it is very clear that the consumer is becoming increasingly involved with the selection of the acute care institution they use.

A comprehensive and more modern definition of the health care marketplace includes third-party payors, the government, physicians, and employers, as well as the individual consumer. In the past, hospitals limited their focus of marketing efforts to the physician. Physicians were considered the major "consumers" of acute care services because they determined almost exclusively where their patients would be admitted, with little direction from third-party payors or the patient. This has drastically changed during the past few years, and it is important that health care institutions acknowledge the increased complexity of the marketplace. To survive in the competitive environment, it is crucial for health care facilities to listen to their consumers.

According to a recent market survey conducted by the National Research Corporation, Lincoln, Nebraska, most consumers would accept a lower quality of care in order to save money.[11] Table 5-8 summarizes some of the consumer preferences the survey identified, and Table 5-9 shows the relative importance of ten different factors in the selection of a hospital to the consumer.

In this new economic environment, it is crucial for an acute care institution to have access to this kind of consumer preference data to make appropriate management decisions, target

Table 5-8   Consumer Preferences for Health Care Services

Consumer's Health Status	Good Quality/ Low Cost (%)	High Quality/ High Cost (%)
Excellent	50	49
Good	53	45
Fair	65	34
Poor	72	24

Table 5-9 Importance of Various Factors in Selecting a Hospital (Rated on a Scale of 1–10, Low–High)

Factor	Rating
Medical staff	9.5
Emergency facilities	9
Nursing staff	9
Complete services	9
New equipment	8.5
Courteous employees	8.5
Pleasant rooms	8.5
Physician recommends	8
Treated there before	7.5
Cost	7.5
Convenience to home	7
Family recommends	6.5
Private rooms	6
Friends recommend	5.5

marketing efforts effectively, and create strategic plans for the future.

EXAMPLE

An institution might be struggling to decide whether it should add capacity to inpatient rooms by adding semi-private rooms at a lower cost or private rooms at higher cost. By having access to marketing research data such as that in Table 5-9, the institution can see that the issue of private rooms is not as important to the customer as pleasant rooms and some other factors. If this same institution has an emergency room that has a poor image and reputation in the community, it could benefit more from investing its resources of time, money, and talent into improving that service rather than spending it on private rooms. Without access to these market research data, the institution might have chosen to improve a service that was not as important to the consumer as the institution believed, and consequently maximum benefit would not be realized from its resources.

After doing a market research study, the organization needs to forecast future hospital market trends based on past and existing trends and consumer values. A hospital can follow this simple methodology to forecast future trends and make effective, appropriate management decisions:

1. Identify the parameters of the hospital's existing or potential service area (external analysis).

2. Gather demographic data for the hospital's existing and potential service area (external analysis).

3. Identify the incidence of various diagnoses based on the demographic data, and project diagnostic trends for the next 10 years.

4. Identify the institution's strengths and weaknesses based on clinical talent, technology, and resources available (internal analysis).

5. Select the specific diagnoses or conditions that match the institution's strengths and weaknesses (strategic plan).

6. Establish programs and health care interventions that match the selected diagnoses in which the hospital has expertise to maximize potential for success and ability to compete in the marketplace (strategic plan).

7. Evaluate and revise strategic plans and programs as needed (operational plan).

DEVELOPING A MARKETING PLAN

A marketing plan is a formal written document that spells out the company's current position, future goals, and objectives for profits and market-share, strategies to obtain the goals, and the tactics that will be used. The following are the main elements of the marketing plan:

1. *Situational analysis*—sometimes referred to as the WOTS-up analysis. The WOTS-up analysis is the acronym for weaknesses, opportunities, threats, and strengths, in the internal and external environment of the organization. (See Chapter 6 for a more detailed description of the WOTS-up analysis.) A company must assess the external environment of the marketplace and the internal strengths and weaknesses of the organization before it can set any future goals.

2. *Marketing goals and objectives*—identifies broad marketing goals and then specific goals and objectives that are measurable and attainable. An example of a marketing goal for a hospital could be to increase market-share of the open heart surgery program. The marketing objective for that goal could be to increase that market-share by 10%.

EXAMPLE

- Marketing goal: The hospital will increase the volume of its open heart surgery program.
- Marketing objective: By October 1, 19X5, the hospital will increase its marketshare of open heart surgeries from 25% to 35%.

---

3. *Marketing strategy*—the methodology the organization will use (*e.g.,* marketing mix, marketing expenditure lev-

els, and marketing allocations) to achieve their predetermined goals and objectives. *Marketing mix* is the specific combination of the four P's (product, price, place, and promotion) that will influence the consumer to buy the product. *Marketing expenditure level* is the percentage of the total budget assigned to the marketing function in an organization. *Marketing allocation* is the amount of resources committed to the marketing of each product, and the amount of resources committed to each function of marketing.

4. *Marketing action plan*—the written component that includes the specific action steps, responsibilities and accountabilities, and time frames for the annual marketing efforts of the company. It is similar to the annual operational plan of an organization but is geared to the action steps for the company's marketing goals.

5. Ongoing *review, evaluation, and revision*—the control function for the marketing plan. It informs management if the plan is being followed and allows for continued evaluation of its appropriateness. In a rapidly changing marketplace, it may be necessary to revise objectives frequently over a year's period of time. This condition is very true for the health care industry of the 1980s.

NEED FOR MARKETING IN HEALTH CARE

All organizations are faced with the problem of producing goods and/or services that will meet the ongoing and changing needs and wants of the marketplace. They are also challenged to increase the market's perception of the value of their goods or services. In the past the health care industry has not, for many reasons, acknowledged or utilized the discipline of marketing to any extent. They did not experience competition to any degree, and marketing was utilized mainly in an environment of competition. Health care was not affected much by demand either. As discussed in Chapter 1, health care services were controlled by the factor of supply because the individual end consumer did not pay for the services. The more services an institution could supply, the more revenue it realized. Institutions paid little attention to what the individual consumer demanded or said about health care products or services.

That trend has significantly changed during the past few years. The Center for Health Management Research, which is the research, development, and educational arm of the Lutheran Hospital Society, conducted a project funded by the W. K. Kellogg Foundation called *Innovations in Health Care Management*.[12] The project identified some of the advanced management practices and characteristics from successful organizations in the business sector. After identifying these traits, the project looked at methods to transfer or adapt these management practices to the health care industry. Two of the 10 most valuable and effective charactistics were foresight and customer-driven products, and have significance for this chapter.

Foresight was defined in the project as a critical awareness and understanding of the changing marketplace for the purpose of looking for potential opportunities and threats in the external environment.

The characteristic of being customer-driven acknowledges that an organization listens and responds to its consumers' needs and wants. One could say that to be consumer-driven is to be concerned with the ultimate goal of marketing. In his article on the social marketing perspective, Seymour Fine identifies marketing as the philosophy that all planning is done with the consumer's needs considered first and foremost.[13] For an acute care institution, this means that needs of physicians, nursing services, contributors, and the organization are all secondary to those of the patient.

Phases in Health Care Marketing Programs

The health care institutions have acknowledged the need for marketing in the past few years. They are at various stages regarding their marketing efforts based on the length of time they have done marketing and the expertise they have within the organization for marketing.

Institutions initially utilize marketing as a promotional or advertising function. This usually happens when the organization first gets started or begins to experience a decline in the sales of their product or service. If business does not increase as a result of these "marketing" efforts, the organization may criticize any marketing efforts as being inefficient and/or a waste of good money.

When marketing efforts have assisted the organization to

survive and have become more sophisticated, the function of marketing changes to one of customer service. The organization usually implements quarantee programs, customer satisfaction surveys, and employee incentives to promote customer satisfaction. As this customer satisfaction function enables continued growth of the company, marketing's attention turns toward new innovations in products and services based on perceived customer wants and needs.

Later on, the organization's marketing efforts focus on increasing the current market-share or percentage of the total business of a particular product or service the company sells in the marketplace. When a company has a high-quality, innovative product or service that is in demand in the marketplace, the only way the organization can grow is to increase its amount of sales of the product in relation to total sales of that same product in the marketplace.

EXAMPLE

A hospital has an excellent open heart surgery program that utilizes the most innovative equipment and techniques. It does about 25% of all the open heart surgeries in a given community. The only way that the program can improve and/or grow is to attempt to do more or, for instance, 50% of all the open heart surgeries in that community. This is an example of an organization in the final phase of its marketing efforts with open heart surgery, trying to improve the program by increasing market position or marketshare.

After having progressed through these phases of a marketing effort, the ultimate phase is usually implemented only by very sophisticated organizations. This phase or function of marketing is the ongoing analysis, planning, and controlling of the organization's opportunities to obtain its goals, while ultimately contributing to the overall quality of life in a society. Many organizations stop short of this phase for various reasons. It is believed that some companies are successful while others fail because they have progressed to this final phase of marketing and have incorporated the goal of contributing to the quality of life into their mission statement.

Implementing Marketing in Health Care

Norman McMillan has outlined the four basic marketing activities usually included in a hospital's marketing program. When the hospital first begins a marketing program, start-up costs traditionally reflect the cost of planning for the marketing effort and for the consumer research activity. According to McMillan, these start-up efforts should be about 1.5% of the total hospital's budget.[14] As the health care institution matures in its marketing efforts, additional expenditures are committed to the activities of design and graphics, public relations, and advertising. The four basic components of the marketing function are outlined in Table 5-10 with budgetary guildelines for all allocation of resources.

It is important to note that the addition of the various marketing functions is a gradual process rather than one that develops overnight. This gradual process is determined by the marketing talent in the organization, the perceptions of top management about the importance of marketing, and the resources available in the organization to accomplish marketing.

It is crucial to the success and effectiveness of marketing efforts that the CEO be committed to listening to the consumer and be comfortable in looking for better ways to do business. As outlined previously, marketing strives to listen to the consumer and then makes changes in the organization's internal environment that might lead to a more satisfied consumer. Health care leaders who feel threatened by change may go through the motions of marketing with few results because of their resistance or discomfort with change. Just as in the private sector, the health care leader of the future will need to be secure enough to rigorously evaluate current operations on an ongoing basis, and to be willing to make changes when neces-

---

Table 5-10 Budgetary Guidelines for Basic Marketing Functions

Marketing Activity	% of Hospital Budget	Definition
Marketing	0.1%	Planning, organizing, and evaluating the total marketing effort.
Consumer research	0.5%	Listening to what the consumer wants and needs for future products and services.
Design and graphics	0.2%	The creation of a solid graphics system.
Public relations and advertising	0.7%	Advertising is paid efforts to communicate or promote a product. Public relations are established relationships in the marketplace to enhance sales of products.

sary for the institution's survival and maintenance of a leadership position in the marketplace.

Leland Kaiser, health care futurist, believes that the ability to respond to the external environment and make necessary changes will be the key concept that determines which health care institutions survive and which ones do not.[15] He believes that a health care provider will need to be able to respond to any environmental factor within 90 days. This means that an institution should be able to make any major decisions regarding a program, service, or product within a 3-month period to be able to respond to opportunities or threats in the environment in a proactive manner. For anyone who has ever worked in a hospital, it is common knowledge that it takes considerably longer than 3 months for most hospitals to make major decisions about services. Reducing the time required to make major decisions usually involves increased risk taking, which, in the past, has not been a very predominant feature of hospital administrations.

MARKETING STRATEGIES FOR NURSING

The profession of nursing, as well as individual nurses, traditionally has not perceived a need to market services. The single most important marketing concept for the nursing profession, as well as the individual nurse, is image. *Image* is the overall impression the consumer or patient has about a product, service, or organization gained through his physical, emotional, and psychological experience.

The image of the nursing profession has been a popular topic in the 1980s. Many seminars and conferences have dealt with the subject. National campaigns have been launched by various nursing organizations to improve the image of nursing.

It is unnecessary to discuss the exact nature of the negative image nursing has had in the past. The more important issue becomes this: What is the image of nursing that is desired? Nurses have demanded the right to be treated "like professionals" in various ways. If nurses want the respect and privileges of professionals, it is important that they display and communicate the image of professionals. Many nursing leaders have varied philosophies regarding how that can and should be accomplished. One method advocated by the author is to utilize marketing principles to communicate that professionalism to the marketplace.

Before outlining a prescriptive model to attain the desired professional image, it is important to consider an additional key point. The consumer's self-image is a very important factor in the field of health marketing. The self-image of an individual is the combination of the way he sees himself and the way he believes others see him. Consumers seek products that have an image consistent with their own self-image. For example, if an individual sees himself as very affluent and sophisticated, he will not shop at a discount store. In the health care setting, if a patient feels he deserves the best of care, he will not seek treatment at a county facility.

Nursing needs to focus more on the self-image of its community of patients. The expectations of potential clients in the community are important to the image nursing receives in the community. Community involvement, networking, and visibility by nursing leaders form a key concept in developing a positive professional image for nursing. A specific marketing plan for nursing services of a health care facility could include these steps:

1. Organize a task force or nursing marketing team to plan the marketing function for the nursing department.

2. Develop a survey tool or interview process for obtaining community perceptions about nursing services and health care needs and wants.

3. Analyze the marketing research data, external threats and opportunities, and internal strengths and weaknesses of the nursing department.

4. Identify the marketing goals and objectives for the nursing department. A marketing goal could be to improve the image of the nursing staff in the community, develop a home health agency or guest relations program.

5. Develop nursing's marketing strategy to attain its goals and objectives. This is the specific methodology (*e.g.*, programs, promotions, resource allocation, etc.) that the nursing department will use to attain its goals and objectives.

6. Develop a plan of action to move the current community image of nursing to the desired image for nursing. Identify action steps, accountabilities, timelines, resources required, promotion, pricing, place, and product.

7. Review, evaluate, and revise goals and objectives and the plan of action as necessary.

Identifying One's Marketing Mix

The individual professional can also take advantage of marketing techniques to promote or advance his or her career. The health care profession is becoming increasingly competitive for the individual. This makes it almost mandatory to gain skills in marketing oneself in order to be successful. Promotions within, as well as outside, the organization depend on the image and visibility displayed by the individual professional in the marketplace. It is possible to utilize the marketing model of the four P's to prescribe a successful marketing regimen to attain individual goals.

Product: The product of the professional is his or her competence, expertise, ability to communicate, problem-solve, lead, teach, make decisions, and manage. The professional decides what resources he or she is willing to spend to develop and improve his product through advanced education, reading, research, and experiences.

Promotion: The professional needs to promote herself/himself through attractive business cards, resumes, business clothes, personal appearance, attitude, publications, and presentations.

Price: The individual needs to identify the "right" price for his services. It could be disastrous to quote a price or salary for services that is too high or too low. The professional must be in touch with the price the market is paying for a like service. The individual needs to then price his or her services higher or lower, based on the image desired.

Place: The old saying, "it's important to be in the right place at the right time" is very appropriate in planning for a successful career. Nurse leaders must work on being visible in the places that will contribute to future professional goals. There are also channels in marketing the individual professional. The professional should identify cost-effective, appropriate channels to "market" his or her services, based on specific goals. Examples of such marketing channels include the following:

- Professional organizations
- Professional offices
- Networking

- Mentor role
- Colleagues
- Community organizations
- Registries
- Past employers
- Executive search firms
- Professional journals

By describing these professional activities in terms of the marketing model of the four P's, it is possible to apply the principles outlined in this chapter to advancing one's career. These key concepts are interpreted in the profession of nursing by some of the following ideas:

1. Actively engage in networking with colleagues (place, promotion).
2. Establish mentor relationships (place, promotion, product).
3. Join professional organizations and volunteer to serve as an officer (promotion).
4. Publish an article (product, promotion).
5. Serve as a reviewer or consultant for a professional journal (promotion).
6. Keep up with the latest professional information by reading many different professional journals (product).
7. Join community organizations to increase visibility and professional image in the community (promotion).
8. Develop presentations for professional organizations and conventions to increase visibility (promotion).
9. Hand out business cards freely (promotion).
10. Develop a firm handshake, good eye contact, and ability to remember names (product, promotion).
11. Develop a positive attitude and professional image (product).
12. Invest in your own growth and development through education and progressive leadership positions (product).
13. Set long- and short-term goals (product).
14. Write a book (promotional, product).
15. Dress for success (product).

16. Exercise regularly to maintain a healthy appearance and attitude and reduce stress (product).

17. Read motivational material (product).

18. Stick with the "winners" (place, promotion).

19. Develop a reputation for integrity (product).

SUMMARY

The discipline of marketing is in its developmental stages in the health care industry and will continue to be an instrumental tool for the survival of the acute care institution of the future. Marketing is the link between society's needs and wants and the marketplace's production of goods and services. Marketing encompasses the exchange process that occurs between the consumer and the producer of goods and services.

The major goals of marketing include maximizing the marketplace's consumption of an organization's products, maximizing consumer satisfaction, and contributing to the quality of life.

A successful marketing program consists of the right combination of these four major components: product, price, promotion, and place or distribution. The proper combination of these four components is called the marketing mix. Price is the most neglected component in health care marketing programs and is driven by the factors of product cost, demand, and competition.

The place or distribution function of marketing includes the factors of distribution channels, locations of distribution, inventory management, and transportation of products. A marketing channel is the set of institutions that perform the function of moving a product from production to consumption. Channels within the distribution systems are called intermediary channels. Direct marketing is a zero-level channel marketing system that has no middleman and in which the producer of goods and services sells directly to the consumer. Most health care services are examples of direct-marketing services.

The components of a formal written marketing plan include a situational analysis, goals and objectives, marketing strategies, action plan and ongoing review, evaluation, and revision. Hospital marketing activities include consumer research, market planning, design and graphics, and public relations and advertising. Developing an effective marketing function in a health care institution is a slow and ongoing process. The various marketing activities are phased in as resources and expertise increase within the organization.

The nurse administrator can benefit on organizational, professional, and personal levels from an understanding and application of the basic marketing principles and practices outlined in this chapter. As competition increases in the health care industry, it will be increasingly important for all health care leaders to possess a working knowledge of marketing techniques to be successful.

REFERENCES

1. Drucker P: Management: Tasks, Responsibilities, Practices. New York, Harper & Row, 1973
2. Kotler P: Marketing Management: Analysis, Planning, and Control. Englewood, NJ, Prentice-Hall
3. Peters T, Waterman: In Search of Excellence. New York, Harper & Row, 1984
4. Bingham R: Economic Concepts. New York, McGraw-Hill, 1984
5. Chadick EG: Product line analysis. Special report #5. American Hospital Association Publication, August 1983
6. Pricing often overlooked in marketing mix. Hospitals, June 16, 1984
7. Henderson BD: Henderson on Corporate Strategy, p 168. Boston, The Boston Consulting Group, 1979
8. Heidingfield MS, Blankenship AB: Marketing, p 199. New York, Barnes and Noble, 1974
9. Ad efforts hike utilization dramatically. Hospitals, June 6, 1984
10. Marketing surge tied to consumers; decision-making muscle being flexed. Hospitals, June 16, 1984
11. Jackson B, Jensen J: Most consumers would accept lower quality hospital care to save money. Modern Healthcare, July 1984
12. Strum D, Coile R: Transferring lessons from high performance organizations. Hospital Forum, May/June 1984
13. Fine S: The health product: A social marketing perspective. Hospitals, June 16, 1984
14. McMillan N: Marketing your hospital: A strategy for survival. American Hospital Publishing, 1981
15. Kaiser L: Survival strategies for non-profit hospitals. Hospital Progress, December 1984

ADDITIONAL READINGS

1. Bezold C: Medical megatrends reshaping delivery and evaluation of care. Modern Healthcare, July 1984
2. Bleeke J: Winning the new competitive game in health care. HFM, December 1982

3. Blendon R: Who will control health care: Seven trends that may determine the future. HMQ
4. Bloom P, Greyser S: The maturing of consumerism. Harvard Business Rev, November-December, 1981
5. Burnett R: Using the market to change health care. Hospitals, September 16, 1984
6. DeWitt C: Getting down to business. Hospitals, October 1, 1981
7. Ellwood P: How competition is reshaping health care. Hospitals, July 16, 1984
8. Evashwick C: Marketing services for seniors. New York, Marketing Long-Term and Senior Care Services, Haworth Press
9. Ginsberg E: Competition in health care: A second opinion. Hospitals, March 16, 1982
10. Holmes P: Competition comes to medical care. Nation's Business, April 1984
11. Seymour D: What PPS means for hospital marketing. Hospitals, June 16, 1984

6

Strategic Planning Methods for Nurses

PRIVATE BUSINESS has used the process of strategic planning to survive in the marketplace since the 1950s. In the mid-1950s, strategic planning was called *long-range planning,* and was done by most large companies. It has been only in the past 5 to 10 years that large hospitals have utilized this planning tool. With the recent changes in government regulations, prospective reimbursement, and contracting for health care services, it has become increasingly important for hospitals to do in-depth planning to survive in a competitive environment. Hospitals that accurately assess their environment, thoroughly identify their strengths, weaknesses, opportunities, and threats, and develop strategic plans will have a better chance of survival.[1]

Nursing has struggled in the past to establish itself as a credible group of health care professionals who have a significant contribution to make in the industry. Being the largest single group of health care professionals in the health care setting, nurses are affected more by the recent changes than are members of any other health care group. It is important, therefore, for nurses to be familar with the management tool of strategic planning, in order to make contributions to the health care organization.

The purpose of this chapter is to describe in simple and succinct language the process, purpose, and benefits of the strategic planning process. By using strategic planning methods, nursing managers can contribute proactively to their institution, their profession, and the health care industry.

The chapter outlines the business model of strategic planning, implemented in an acute care setting. In the current environment of cost containment in health care, nurse managers will merely move from one crisis to another, if they ignore the planning component of effective management. To function effectively, each nurse manager should have a practical understanding and "hands-on" working knowledge of the strategic planning process. The use of this process will allow nurses to feel they have control over the future of their profession, as well as input into their institution's future goals and the health care delivery system.

This chapter is intended to be of assistance to nurse managers with little or no business background. The examples and how to's are geared specifically for the nursing division in a health care institution. Knowledge of the process will enable nurse managers to identify effectively the direction the nursing division will take and actively contribute meaningful data to the institution's strategic plan.

OBJECTIVES

After completion of this chapter, the reader will be able to

1. Outline the strategic planning process.
2. Identify two reasons for doing strategic planning.
3. Develop measurable objectives for an acute care institution.
4. Develop a mission statement for a hospital.
5. Describe the format of a strategic plan.
6. Develop a WOTS-up analysis.
7. Develop and implement operational objectives that accomplish the goals of a strategic plan.

DEFINITION OF STRATEGIC PLANNING

The management function of planning is not new to nurse administrators and managers. To plan is to make the decision to go in a specific direction, and then allocate organizational resources to proceed in that direction. Very simply, planning can be broken down into short-range or operational planning, and long-range or strategic planning. The major focus of this chapter is the use of long-range or strategic planning in health care, to accomplish predetermined goals in a health care setting.

Strategic planning is defined as the formulation and implementation of strategies to accomplish specific organizational goals.[2] The process begins with an indepth analysis of the current environment, internal strengths and weaknesses of the organization, and external opportunities and threats in the environment, for the purpose of setting appropriate and realistic goals. After organizational goals are identified, specific objectives and strategies to accomplish those goals can be determined.

Strategic planning is long-range planning that extends from 3 to 5 years into the future. Strategic planning incorporates an extensive analysis of the internal and external environment of the organization to determine constraints, realistic goals, and resources necessary to pursue a specific direction.

The final product of the strategic planning process allows more effective decision making and efficient use and control of resources, and assists the organization in directing all of its efforts toward its predetermined goals. Strategic planning minimizes the risks for an organization and allows the organization to take advantage of opportunities in the environment. The opportunities for the organization are identified in the environmental analysis.

Strategic planning goals and objectives are more generic and less specific than those in operational planning. They are developed and flow from the values or mission statement of the leadership of the organization. A mission statement for an organization is a broad statement of its values or reason for existence.[4] The following is a sample mission statement and goals for a nursing department.

SAMPLE MISSION AND GOAL STATEMENTS FOR NURSING

Mission Statement

The Department of Nursing will deliver quality, cost-effective, patient care, promote professional practice, and make significant contributions to the institution and the nursing profession.

Goals

   I. Develop, maintain, and improve programs, services, and operations to ensure quality patient care, while encouraging staff participation.

  II. Promote and further develop an atmosphere and systems that achieve professional practice.

 III. Reduce costs and increase revenue in a coordinated manner while maintaining standards of care.

 IV. Create, maintain, and evaluate programs to ensure development of nursing staff.

  V. Achieve recognition for the nursing department by making significant contributions to the institution and the nursing profession through research and marketing.

There are essentially four major salient points of strategic planning that can assist the reader in understanding strategic planning[5]:

1. Strategic planning deals with the future impact of current events and trends. It looks at the cause/effect consequences of planned decisions over a period of time. It considers alternate courses of action that exploit opportunities and avoid threats to the organization.

2. Strategic planning is process-oriented, and is a continuous, flexible, and integral function of management.

3. Strategic planning is a management attitude and requires a conscious commitment and decision to do it right.

4. Strategic planning is a system that links the three levels of management planning. These three levels of management planning include the following:

   - Long-range or strategic planning
   - Medium-range or program planning
   - Short-range or operational planning

After considering these important facts about strategic planning, a comprehensive definition follows:

> Strategic planning is the systematic effort of a hospital to establish basic purposes, objectives, policies, and strategies, and develop detailed plans to implement policies and strategies to attain the hospital's purpose and objectives.[6]

> Program or medium-range planning is the part of strategic planning that determines the programs and/or services that should be provided by the hospital to attain the hospital's purpose. Program planning is sometimes called administrative planning.

> Operational or short-range planning is the determination of budgets, allocation of staff, and establishment of productivity standards, and so on, on an annual basis.

It is important to note that goals in strategic planning should be appropriate for a 3- to 5-year period. If a goal is not appropriate after a year, it is either an operational goal or a specific objective in the strategic plan.

OPERATIONAL OR SHORT-TERM PLANNING

The most common type of planning that nurse managers do is short-range or operational planning. Operational planning is the setting of annual or short-term goals and objectives. The operational planning process usually takes place a few months prior to the beginning of the institution's fiscal year and is done in conjunction with budgeting. Operational planning involves the development of departmental goals and objectives for the coming year. The budget is the financial commitment to obtain the specific goals and objectives that are identified by management. Operational goals are usually broken down into maintenance goals and improvement goals. *Maintenance goals* represent specific organizational standards that are maintained from one year to the next. Examples of such maintenance goals include the following:

- Compliance with predetermined productivity standards
- Compliance with revenue and expense guidelines
- Patient care plan compliance
- Compliance with the predetermined turnover goals
- Compliance with predetermined patient satisfaction survey target results
- Compliance with a predetermined medication error percentage

Operational plans for a unit or department also include objectives for improvement of services. Improvement objectives include capital equipment purchases, new services, procedures, and programs that would increase productivity, efficiency, or services. Examples of such improvement objectives include the following:

1. Develop two new programs to meet community needs by January 1, 19x3 at a cost of $10,000 per program.
2. Purchase a new nurse call system by October 1, 19x2 for less than $100,000 to improve response time to patients.
3. By December 30, 19x3 develop, implement, and evaluate hospital-wide policies and procedures to effectively care for patients suffering from AIDS.
4. Develop and implement a market research survey to identify unmet community health care needs and services by June 30, 19x2.

As mentioned previously, strategic planning is long-range planning, whereas operational planning is short-range planning. The differences between strategic planning and operational planning are outlined in Table 6-1.

HISTORICAL PERSPECTIVE

The business or private sector has been doing strategic planning for at least the past 10 to 15 years. Initially, only large corporations invested the necessary human and fiscal resources to accomplish this sophisticated process. Later on, smaller companies implemented this management planning tool. Over the past 5 years, hospitals have begun to use the strategic planning process. As a result of increased competition arising out of deregulation in health care, hospitals are adopting more business-

Table 6-1 Operational Planning vs. Strategic Planning

Criteria	Operational	Strategic
Timeframe	1 Year	3–5 Years
Responsibility	Middle management	Top management
Goals	Specific, measurable goals and objectives	Broad, ongoing, generic goals
Purpose	Plan and control yearly operations	Set direction, maximize organization's ability to respond to a changing environment
Procedure	Accomplished by department on yearly basis	Accomplished by the combined efforts of entire organization and updated yearly

oriented approaches to the management of their organizations. There was a time when hospitals were managed by physicians or religious orders, and little attention was given to specific management, financial, or business skills.

As the complexity of the health care industry increased, it became apparent that health care institutions could not fulfill their mission "to care for the sick" if they could not manage their resources efficiently. This insight led to more "business-oriented" hospital administrators. The increased complexity of the field also led to the establishment and growth of health administration programs at the bachelor's and master's level on college campuses.

The strategic planning process is one tool that allows the organization to take an objective look at its strengths, weaknesses, present situation, and projected future, to determine a realistic and desired course of action for attaining future goals. Health care managers must take the responsibility of equipping themselves with the management tools that can assist them in accomplishing their desired goals and future. It is believed that by understanding and utilizing the strategic planning process nurse managers can significantly contribute to the health care delivery system and the practice of professional nursing.

GOAL SETTING FOR THE PLANNING PROCESS

Yogi Berra summarized the importance of goal setting when he said, "If you don't know where you are going, you'll probably end up somewhere else."

Without goals, long- or short-range, the individual uses

energy very inefficiently. Efforts are diluted by the constant changing of direction. Without goals, an individual or organization has little insight into past successes. The measurement for success is lacking because there is no end-point or goal to measure progress.

Goal setting is the most important step in planning. However, before setting goals, an individual or organization needs to first look at "where they are" and then "where they want to be." Planning bridges the gap between "where you are" and "where you want to be." By identifying these two points, all energy can be channeled to the shortest path between the points.

Only 5% of the population uses goal-setting techniques in their daily lives. Of this 5%, 95% achieve their goals. These statistics certainly plead the case for the value of goal setting as a tool and measure of success.

Goal setting at the organizational level is defined as the desired state that a system is attempting to achieve by planning, organizing, and controlling. The goals are created by the leaders in the organization. Specifically, for a health care organization, these goals are identified by the administrative team and governing board.[3]

Effective goal setting involves a measure of vision and risk taking. *Vision* refers to the ability to set goals that are not limited to what is presently inevitable. In order to be meaningful, goals must stretch the imagination and efforts of the individual or organization setting them. If goals are inevitable occurrences in the future, they are set too low and are no real measure of progress or accomplishment. According to Dr. Robert H. Schuller, founder of the $20 million Crystal Cathedral in Garden Grove, California, "If future goals are determined by existing resources, they are set too low." Dr. Schuller set a goal to build a one-of-a-kind drive-in, walk-in church with resources totalling only $400. If he had set long-range goals based on his then existing resources, the Crystal Cathedral would never have become a goal, let alone a reality. Therefore, vision is a critical asset for managers involved in the goal setting and long-range planning for an organization.

A second critical factor in goal setting is the ability to take calculated risks. Any goal worth achieving holds the possibility of failure or success. When a leader has a great vision for goal setting but lacks the ability to risk possible failure, the goal is never shared or never dared. If the goal is never declared, there is no chance of attaining it. When the leader cannot risk sharing the goal with others, the group cannot support him in the attainment of that goal.

In conclusion, it is vital that the institution's leadership possess a sense of vision and the ability to take calculated risks for the forward movement and goal attainment of the organization.

The Need for Strategic Planning

The importance of strategic planning for health care institutions and nursing administrators has grown rapidly in the past few years. The major reason for this increase in importance is the rapidly changing health care environment. Managers in the business sector have found that by identifying the mission of their company and developing specific strategies to accomplish their mission, they could give more direction to their organizations. Managers and organizations can better respond to competition and a changing environment, if they have developed a strategic planning mentality.

In the past, health care institutions were in the business of simply caring for sick people. Their mission statement, although rarely formally identified, was just that: "To care for the sick." A hospital's strategy for providing services was simply to wait for sick people to be admitted to the institution. A few institutions did have marketing plans to increase patient census. However, the plans usually consisted of merely buying the latest medical equipment requested by physicians, and providing social events, meals, and medical suites on campus for the medical staff. These marketing efforts were usually quite effective, because the physician was considered the main client of the institution.

However, times have changed. The health care environment is more closely approximating the competitive private sector. Hospitals are feeling increased pressure to adopt more business-like methods of operating. In the very near future, hospitals that do not adopt a more formal process of long-range planning will not be able to compete with institutions that do.

Another factor increasing the need for strategic planning in all organizations in the 1980s is the faster pace of life and changes in general. In the past, managers could operate similarly from one year to the next. This, however, is no longer the case. In the health care industry, it is difficult for managers to keep up with the latest changes, let alone plan for those changes.

Hospitals have traditionally acted or reacted with minimal consideration for the long-term consequences of their actions. This is why hospitals have the reputation for using a "crisis-management" style. As an oversimplified example, nursing "solved" the nursing shortage about 25 years ago by introducing the 2-year associate degree program. Now, however, nursing faces the "entry to practice" issue as a consequence of that solution. Because of that short-range solution, there are currently three different entry levels to the profession of nursing: diploma, associate degree, and baccalaureate. Strategic planning may not have avoided this problem, but the strategic planning process forces the leadership to assess the present situation and set goals considering future threats and opportunities. In many instances, indepth assessment, analysis, and planning minimize the potential problems resulting from crisis-oriented short-range decision making.

The Purpose of Strategic Planning

Too often, the purpose of planning is not clearly understood by managers, and, therefore, planning is perceived as merely "extra work." When managers are aware of the relationship between the economic realities of the external environment and their personal and organizational goals and objectives, they have an appreciation for the effectiveness of strategic planning as a management tool.[7] In the past, nursing has identified what it had a lot of or what it wanted to do, and then planned goals and objectives along those lines. In the present health care environment, the successful nurse leaders will be those who identify the need for specific health care services, and then plan and allocate resources to meet those needs. It can be said that one of the major purposes of strategic planning is to identify the needs for health care services of the hospital's target market and to formulate specific goals and objectives to meet those needs. Identifying specific client-centered health care needs and meeting them is the key to survival for health care organizations in the future.

Another major purpose of strategic planning is to establish a common data base for an organization. Before realistic goals and objectives can be identified, the organization must know where it is and where it wants to go. The following are the basic questions requiring answers to develop a common data base [4]:

1. What does the organization believe?
2. What is valued?
3. Where is the organization now?
4. What are the organization's strengths and weaknesses?
5. What are the potential threats and opportunities in the environment?
6. Where does the organization want to go?
7. How can the organization get there?
8. What is the long-range plan?
9. What is the short-range plan?

These simple questions can be translated into a goal-setting model that parallels the strategic planning model. Figure 6-1 shows these respective models.

Once the strategic plan has been developed, it can be used to develop yearly operational plans. Specific operational goals and objectives can be identified easily and flow from the broad goals that continue from one year to the next. After accom-

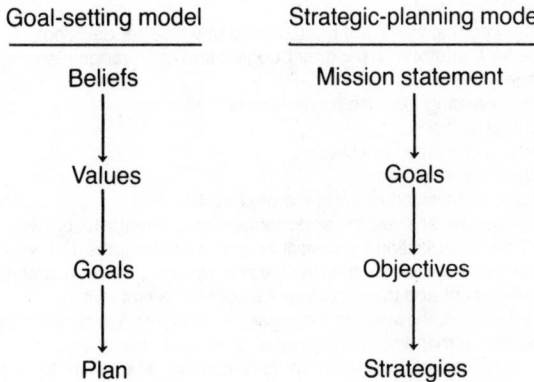

Figure 6-1. *Goal setting compared with strategic planning.*

plishing this process, the organization can then make decisions as to how it will allocate resources to various units and/or programs within the organization. Allocation of resources will follow programs that conform with the goals and mission statement. The strategic planning process can ensure, therefore, that resources will be attached to well-thought-out goals and objectives. This should maximize efficiency and the contribution of resources to the preestablished goals and objectives of the organization. When the strategic planning process is used, resources will be allocated only to projects and programs contributing to the predetermined goals and direction of the organization. Table 6-2 outlines various reasons for implementing strategic planning in an organization.

THE PROCESS OF STRATEGIC PLANNING

The process of strategic planning is also called the "plan to plan." The plan to plan includes all the steps, from making a commitment to do strategic planning to the actual completion

---

Table 6-2   Rationale for Implementing Strategic Planning

1. Give direction to the organization.
2. Accelerate and improve efficiency of the organization.
3. Weed out poor, underutilized services.
4. Flush out strategic issues for top management consideration.
5. Concentrate resources on important services.
6. Guide divisions and research team in developing new services and programs that are needed.
7. Develop better information for top managers to make better decisions.
8. Develop a better frame of reference for budgets and short-range planning.
9. Teach managers to plan.
10. Provide mind-expanding exercise for managers.
11. Gain control of operations.
12. Develop better coordination of activities.
13. Eliminate duplication of efforts.
14. Develop better communication within the organization.
15. Develop a situational analysis of opportunities and threats to provide a better awareness of the organization's potential in light of its strengths and weaknesses.
16. Develop a sense of security among managers, resulting from understanding the changing environment and the department's ability to adapt to it.
17. Provide a road map to show where the organization is going and how to get there.
18. Set more realistic, demanding, yet attainable goals and objectives.
19. Review and audit present activities to enable easy adaptation to a changing environment.
20. Assess success of organization in goal attainment.

of the tangible strategic plan. There are several different approaches to accomplish the strategic planning process[3]:

1. The *top-down method* is implemented when the strategic plan is developed by the top administrative team and simply shared with the hospital staff. This approach is commonly implemented in a centralized organization.

2. The *bottom-up method* involves department managers in developing goals and objectives, and then the top administrative team develops the formal strategic plan.

3. A *combination of top-down and bottom-up methods* uses two-way communication techniques to develop the strategic plan. This method is used in large, decentralized organizations. The top administrative team identifies the broad goals and values of the organization and then calls on the department managers to develop goals that coincide with the broad institutional goals.

4. The *team planning method* uses a team or task force to obtain input from administration and staff within the organization to develop a strategic plan. The team or task force actually develops or writes the plan, but it is based totally on input from all levels of the organization.

In each of these methods, the process of developing the formal strategic plan involves the same specific steps.Figure 6-2 shows a model of the basic strategic planning process. Each step in the process is described in detail below:

Step 1—The first and most important step in strategic planning is obtaining a commitment by top administration to develop a strategic plan. This step is the foundation for the effective development and implementation of the strategic planning function in an organization. If commitment from the top administrator is lacking, the process will be a formality rather than a productive management effort.

Step 2—The education of managers on the "how to's" and "whys" of strategic planning is a very important step for an organization to implement before attempting to do a strategic plan. This is a crucial step in the process because if managers do not understand the benefits of planning and how to do it, they will perceive the process as "busy work" and will be resistant and uncooperative. Health care managers currently are faced with many challenges and demands. They need to be informed and educated in how this management tool can make their jobs more organized and goal directed.

Step 3—The next step in the planning process involves

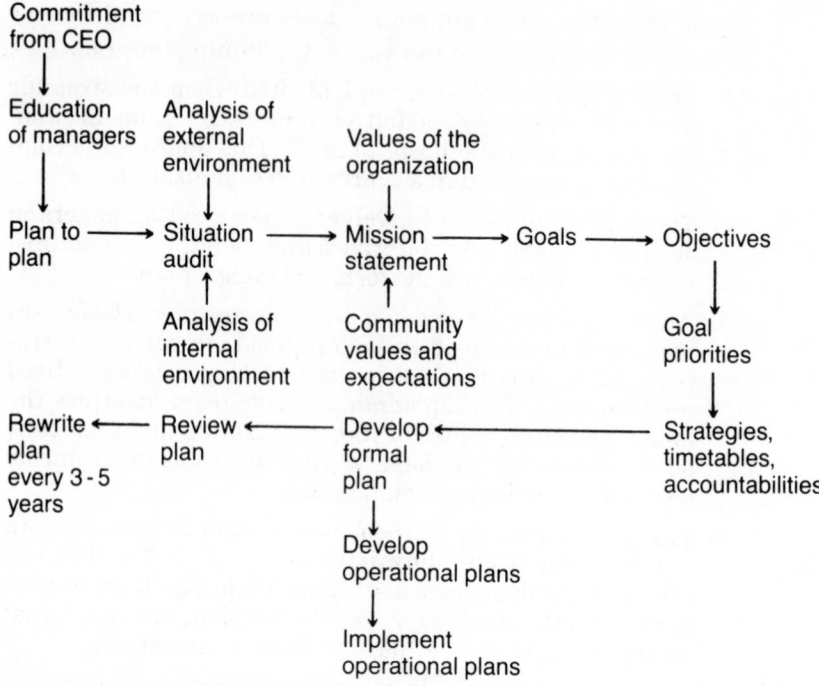

Figure 6-2. *Steps in strategic-planning process.*

doing an environmental assessment or situation audit. This step can be performed by the top management team, the planning department, or an outside consultant. The environmental assessment analyzes the marketplace for forces and trends that are currently affecting the organization, as well as for the forces and trends that will affect the organization in the future. The environmental assessment includes a WOTS-up analysis. WOTS-up is an acronym for the weaknesses, opportunities, threats, and strengths of the organization. After these factors are identified, the organization can begin to set some realistic goals.[1]

Step 4—The mission statement is the next component to be developed. The mission statement is usually developed by the top management team in collaboration with the governing board. The mission statement is a broad statement that describes the organization's purpose, values, and reason for existence.

Step 5—Broad organization goals are then set by top management. These goals are broad, long-range, ongoing goals of the organization that extend at least 3 to 5 years into the future.

Step 6—Next, departmental objectives and strategies are developed by managers and staff for each department. These objectives and goal must fit in with the broad organizational goals.

Step 7—Next, the top administrative team prioritizes and approves departmental objectives and strategies, based on the available resources of the organization. Some of the department goals may need to be held over for the next year, if there are not enough organizational resources to implement all the desired goals in a particular year.

Step 8—Accountabilities and timelines are determined for the goals and objectives. It is very important to assign an individual to be accountable for each specific goal, and place that person's name alongside the goal. When groups of individuals are assigned accountability for a goal, it is difficult to hold anyone accountable.

Step 9—The formal strategic plan is written. Here again, it is difficult for a "group" or team to write a plan, and so one individual is usually assigned the responsibility of putting everyone's input into the appropriate format. In most organizations, after the plan is completed, it is reviewed and formally voted on by the governing body.

Step 10—The strategic plan is reviewed, updated, and revised on an annual basis. This is a very important step, not to be overlooked, because of the rapid changes currently occurring in the health care industry. As regulations change and competition increases, it is vital that the organization reevaluate its environment and determine if the assumptions that the strategic plan are built on still hold true.

Step 11 — The strategic plan is rewritten after 3 to 5 years. With the current rate of change, it may be necessary to rewrite the strategic plan more frequently in the future.

The Environmental Assessment or Situation Audit

The first step in the strategic planning process is the environmental assessment or situation audit. This is an analysis of past, current, and future data that have impacted or could impact the organization. It is important to acknowledge where the organization has been and where it currently is to make appropriate management decisions about the future. Assessment of future data can be obtained by various forecasting techniques. Specific forecasting techniques are discussed in detail in Chapter 7.

The situation audit contains five major components[3]:

1. Past performance of the organization
2. Current situation of the organization
3. Future forecasts for the organization
4. Expectations from outside interests
5. Expectations from inside interests

The level of analysis for a situational audit is determined by the resources available to the organization. The resources determining this level of sophistication include financial resources, time, the planning expertise of management, and the commitment by the CEO.

The major purpose of the situation audit is to identify and analyze driving trends and influences on the organization in order that appropriate management and organizational strategies can be implemented to assist the organization in the accomplishment of its goals.

The data base created from the situation audit can include the analysis of many different factors and/or parameters in the environment from past, present, and future perspectives. The level of sophistication of this data analysis, again, depends on available resources.

A typical data base for a health care organization could include these parameters[3]:

- Revenue from patient services
- Net profit from operations
- Market share
- Cash flow
- Capital expenditures
- Long-term debt
- Available organizational resources
- The community's perceptions of the service
- Patient satisfaction indices
- Program development
- Marketing efforts
- Outreach programs
- Productivity
- Labor relations status

- Organizational restructuring
- Foundation performance
- Competition
- Status of existing technology

The following are some sample questions requiring answers when a comprehensive data base is being developed [3]:

1. Who are the organization's consumers?
2. What market is the organization in?
3. Where do the hospital's consumers come from?
4. How many consumers are repeat consumers?
5. Is the hospital's technology static or dynamic?
6. What share of the market does the organization have?
7. Is the market seasonal?
8. How do consumers perceive the quality, service, and cost of the organization's products?

A comprehensive analysis of the organization's resources must be made before any specific goals or objectives are identified. Organizational resources determine the goals the organization can accomplish realistically. The important resources that require analysis include the following:

- Financial resources
- Employee skills, productivity, and turnover
- The facility's capacity and technology
- The potential for new program development
- Managerial performance, leadership capabilities, personnel development, and planning

An analysis of the environment of the organization is crucial to its ability to plan realistic goals. The environmental factors that demand consideration in a comprehensive environmental assessment include the following[3]:

- Economic factors and trends
- Demographic characteristics of clients
- Social factors of community, clients
- Political trends, associations, threats
- Technology of competition and of the future
- Legal threats and potentials
- Changing values and ethics

Table 6-3 shows a sample format that could be used to compile the criteria data for establishing the organization's data base for its situation audit.

WOTS-UP ANALYSIS

As previously mentioned, the WOTS-up analysis is an acronym for the weaknesses, opportunities, threats, and strengths of the organization.[3] An effective method for developing a WOTS-up analysis begins with a blank worksheet as shown in Figure 6-3. This worksheet can be used by the planning committee, department directors, and/or the top administrative team for brainstorming. Participants in this activity are encouraged to write down all their ideas without censoring their responses. The more responses obtained, the better the analysis will be. The chairman of the planning committee, CEO, and/or director of planning can decide which responses are appropriate for the purposes of the organization and which of the ideas will be eliminated from the formal plan.

The process of objectively looking at the strengths and weaknesses of the organization is crucial to an accurate assessment of where the organization currently is, as well as to what it can realistically accomplish. Individual managers may hesitate at first to identify strengths and weaknesses of their departments because of the implications this has for their own

Table 6-3 Data Base for Situation Audit

Criteria	Past	Present	Future
Customers			
Marketshare			
Competition			
Environment			
Economic			
Demographic			
Social			
Political			
Technological			
Legal			
Organization's resources			
Financial			
Human			
Plant and equipment			
Services			
Management			

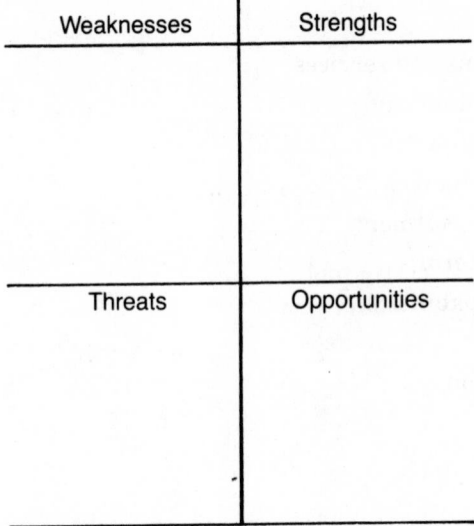

Weaknesses	Strengths
Threats	Opportunities

Figure 6-3. *WOTS-up analysis worksheet.*

performances. However, after being involved in a WOTS-up analysis a few times, managers become more comfortable with the process and learn how to objectively assess their department's strengths and weaknesses.

The kinds of factors important for a health care organization to consider in the WOTS-up analysis include the following:

Weaknesses and Strengths

1. Financial position
2. Cashflow position
3. Marketing efforts
4. Expertise of administrative team
5. Expertise of department managers
6. Productivity
7. Clinical expertise of staff
8. Medical staff expertise
9. Plant and equipment
10. Programs and services (quality of)
11. Location
12. Marketshare

Opportunities

1. New programs and services
2. Improved technology
3. Population growth
4. Legislative changes
5. Physician recruitment
6. Referral patterns
7. Planning capabilities
8. New markets
9. Diversification

Threats

1. Competition
2. Legislative changes
3. Litigation
4. Staffing shortages
5. Environmental disasters
6. Increased regulations
7. Decreasing demand for services
8. Unionization of employees
9. Decreasing reimbursement
10. Increase in accounts receivables
11. Loss of accreditation
12. Decrease in patient satisfaction

Components of the Strategic Plan

After completing the situation audit and the environmental assessment, the management team can focus on the actual components of the formal plan, which include the following:

1. Mission statement
2. Organizational goals
3. Organizational objectives
4. Strategies to obtain objectives
5. Timeframes
6. Required resources
7. Accountabilities

The specific components of any organization's strategic plan varies somewhat based on the resources available for and committed to planning, as well as the backgrounds of the planners. Each of these generic components will be explained in detail, complete with examples for a health care setting.

MISSION STATEMENT AND BROAD GOALS

The *mission statement* is a broad statement that describes the organization's overall purpose or its reasons for existence. The mission statement sets the direction or goals of the organization. The mission statement is the company's philosophy or creed and is considered the cornerstone of the company.[4] This mission statement is determined frequently by the values and goals of the top administrator or founder. All of the goals, objectives, policies, programs, and services are rooted or founded on this mission statement or philosophy.

Mission statements determine many facets of the organization and are important in evaluating the organization's success or failure. Components of a health care organization that are determined by its mission statement include the following:

- The nature of the programs and services the institution provides and will develop in the future
- The potential size and scope of the organization
- The clients who will be serviced
- The organization's response to competition
- The diversification efforts of the organization

Mission statements are purposefully vague and broad in their nature so they may endure environmental changes and allow the organization to respond to the changes yet remain within the realm of its mission. Mission statements should be able to survive for as long as 10 years and still be appropriate. Some organizations develop mission statements that are rather short and describe the overall purpose of the organization. A few of these short sample mission statements are as follows:

SAMPLE SHORT MISSION STATEMENTS

- The XYZ Hospital is dedicated to meeting all the health care needs of the community in a cost-effective manner.
- The XYZ Medical Center is dedicated to the research, education, and care of cancer patients.

Other health care organizations include some of their broad, ongoing goals in their mission statements. These more comprehensive mission statements can include the socioeconomic purpose of the organization, thrusts and characteristics of the insitution, managerial practices, relationship to the community and medical staff, markets served, and programs and/or services provided. An example of such a comprehensive expanded mission statement follows:

SAMPLE LONG MISSION STATEMENT

The XYZ Hospital is dedicated to
- Providing a full-range of health care services for the entire community, regardless of ability to pay.
- Maintaining its 12% marketshare position in the community.
- Supporting of ongoing medical and nursing inhouse education via residency programs and nursing school affiliations.
- Providing cost-effective quality medical and nursing care.
- Maintaining state-of-the-art technology in the organization.
- Maintaining an innovative, participative approach to management of the organization.

In organizations that use the shortened form of a mission statement, the additional statements in the long mission statement above are considered ongoing organizational goals. An organizational goal is a broad, abstract statement that is open-ended. A goal does not have a timeframe and may never be fully accomplished, hence their ongoing nature.[4] An example of a shortened generic mission statement for a hospital with broad ongoing goals follows:

MISSION STATEMENT

XYZ Hospital is dedicated to meeting all the health care needs of the community in a cost-effective manner.

Broad Ongoing Goals

- Goal 1: The hospital will provide a full range of services to the community, regardless of ability to pay.
- Goal 2: The hospital will maintain its market position.
- Goal 3: The hospital will support ongoing medical and nursing education.
- Goal 4: The hospital will maintain state of the art technology for provision of health care services.
- Goal 5: The hospital is committed to providing an innovative, participative environment for managers of the organization.
- Goal 6: The hospital will provide quality medical and nursing care to all patients.

ORGANIZATONAL OBJECTIVES

An objective is a specific program and/or method to accomplish a broad ongoing organizational goal. An objective has a time-frame, has an ending point, and can be measured. Objectives are very specific and concrete in comparison with broad, ongoing organizational goals.[4]

Steiner identifies ten major characteristics of objectives that need to be kept in mind when writing objectives for an organization[3]:

1. An objective must be suitable for achieving the organization's mission and goals. All objectives should be relevant to the specific goals or purposes of the organization.

2. Objectives most be measurable over time and be quantifiable in concrete terms.

3. Objectives should be possible to achieve, or feasible.

4. Objectives should be acceptable to people within the organization, so that they receive support and can be realistically accomplished.

5. Objectives should be flexible yet firm. They should be capable of being modified when unforseen problems arise.

6. Objectives should be stated in a simple, succinct manner, so they are *understandable*. If they are too complicated to understand, they will never be attained.

7. Objectives should receive *commitment* from managers who are assigned to accomplish them or who develop them. Commitment is essential for accomplishment.

8. Objectives should be developed through staff participation. When staff are involved in developing objectives, there is a stronger commitment to their accomplishment.

9. Objectives must be linked to the organizational mission, purpose, and broad goals.

10. Objectives should motivate employees to action. They should force staff to stretch beyond themselves, and not be too easy or too hard.

STRATEGIES

Strategies are specific methods of accomplishing organizational goals and objectives. Strategies include the specific program that is developed to meet a goal or objective. For example, if an organization has an objective of developing a home health program, the strategies it might utilize to accomplish this objective might include the following:

- Identify the specific need for the program through a market research survey.
- Identify a specific individual to be responsible for developing a business plan for the program.
- Investigate the possibility of a joint venture with the local hospital.
- Attend an educational presentation on "How To Start A Hospital-Based Home Health Program."

TIMEFRAMES

Timeframes are deadlines that are identified to accomplish a strategy in the strategic plan. Timeframes are important to identify because they create a sense of urgency and force action on an issue. Without identifying deadlines, little action or follow through on a plan would occur as a result of the tendency for procrastination.

REQUIRED RESOURCES

Required resources are included by strategy to formally match scarce resources to specific strategies. When strategies are not considered in relation to the resources that are needed, the commitment is a weak one at best. In an environment where resources are decreasing on an ongoing basis, it is important to identify the magnitude and type of resources that are required to attain each strategy in the long-range plan.

ACCOUNTABILITIES

Accountability is held by the person responsible for seeing that a strategy is actually implemented. Only individuals can be accountable for steps or strategies in a plan. Groups of individuals are not the most effective way to identify accountabilities because members can each blame the others for failure to follow through. If a group is truly responsible, the chairman or group leader needs to be listed as the accountable person to maximize effectiveness of follow through.

PARTICIPANTS IN THE PLANNING PROCESS

The major leadership role and responsibility for strategic planning lies with the chief executive officer (CEO).[3] There are two types of management responsibilities for planning. There is the responsibility for planning and managing organizational strategies that determine the direction the company chooses to take. This responsibility lies with the CEO. The other type of responsibility is the planning and management of daily operations. The responsibility for operations is ultimately the CEO's. However, in many decentralized organizations responsibility for operations may be delegated to others.

The responsibility for strategic management lies soley on the shoulders of the CEO. Therefore, it is key for effective strategic planning that there is a strong commitment by the CEO to this concept and process. Peter Drucker explains the prime task of strategic planning by top management in his popular text, *Management: Tasks, Responsibilites, and Practices.* The prime task of strategic planning by top management is the "task of thinking through the mission of the business, that is, of asking the question, what is our business and what should it be?"[8] This leads to the setting of objectives, the development of strategies and plans, and the marketing of today's decisions for tommorrow's results. Clearly, this can be done only by a role in the organization that can see the entire business, that can make decisions affecting the entire business, that can balance objectively the needs of today against the needs of tommorrow, and that can allocate resources of men and money to obtain results.[8]

The participants in the strategic planning process are key for the success of the endeavor. Each group of participants in the process needs to take its role and responsibility seriously for the overall success of the planning process for the organization.

Table 6-4 outlines the roles and responsibilities of all participants in the hospital strategic planning process.

BENEFITS OF STRATEGIC PLANNING

The major benefit of strategic planning is the establishment of a keen sense of direction for the organization. This benefit is paramount to all other benefits. The long-term use of strategic planning ensures some continuity of direction over time. The viability of multi-staged projects or programs requiring more than one year to accomplish are carried over from one year to the next by the strategic plan. The phases of long projects are

Table 6-4 Roles and Responsibilities in Strategic Planning

Participants	Responsibilities
Governing board	Determines planning policy. Hires CEO. Represents the community. Ultimate decision maker.
CEO	Sets the climate for planning. Must be actively involved. Reports to Board. Has organizational responsibility for planning and process. Delegates planning work.
Planning committee (optional)	Reports to governing board. Has planning expertise. Consultants to department heads on technical matters and directs planning function. Makes recommendations to governing board.
Department heads	Develop program and operational planning objectives. Provide technical expertise on specific problems/opportunities. Monitor results and the attainment of operational objectives. Implement programs and objectives in their areas. Provide ongoing feedback to top administrative team.
Medical staff	Serve on specific committees. Provide technical expertise. Support proposed programs and services.
Adhoc committees	Complete tasks as assigned. Make reports to planning committee and top administrative team.

carried over from one operational plan to another through the use of the strategic plan.

Similarly, when the organization has a strategic plan to guide its efforts, there is a minimal amount of disruption in the accomplishment of goals during times of management or leadership turnover. The strategic plan ensures continuity from one year to another even though the initiators of the plan may have left the institution.

While the strategic plan ensures continuity of direction, it is both flexible and adaptable to a changing environment. Because of the in-depth environmental assessment and analysis that is done, sophisticated forms of the process include contingency plans. The plan is also reviewed, revised, and updated on a yearly basis. This is usually adequate to maintain its functional value.

The indepth strategic planning process is done every 3 to 5 years to maintain a current data base for making quality decisions and identify realistic goals. Yearly operational planning utilizes this data base for specific departmental goal setting and resource utilization. This is a more cost-effective use of information than having to regenerate it every year.

The long-range planning function benefits nursing managers in various ways. It avoids managing in the "crisis mode," and therefore decreases the manager's stress level. It increases managerial confidence by planning and making decisions in an environment that is not filled with emotion and time constraints. Decision making tends to be more logical and less emotional when not done in a crisis mode. Strategic planning minimizes the risk and uncertainties for the organization while the manager's confidence in his ability to manage all situations is increased.

The format of strategic planning includes a detailed assessment of the organization's weaknesses and strengths for the purpose of determining realistic goals. This process encourages the practice of objectively looking at individual and organizational strengths and weaknesses to seek improvement. Once this process is accepted, managers tend to be less defensive in analyzing their department's strengths and weaknesses in other contexts. Such insight into one's own functional area can only improve the organization's performance and productivity.

BARRIERS TO STRATEGIC PLANNING

The benefits of long-range planning clearly outweigh the barriers, but some do exist. The strategic planning process is a new process for health care managers, involving new terminology and processes. There is frequently an increase in anxiety in learning a new function. If the educational component for the process, or the leadership is not adequate, anxiety will escalate and result in resistance to the process.[10] There must be a clear, firm commitment to the process and active participation from the CEO for it to be successful. Ultimate responsibility and accountability for the strategic planning process in any organization is with top management. If nursing administration does not understand or accept the importance and significance of the process, there will be resistance from nursing managers. Commitment from top management is crucial and cannot be stressed enough.

In an economic environment that is striving to be more cost effective, there will be many managers who feel they cannot afford to implement long-range planning. However, managers with the vision and commitment to take charge of their destiny and make significant contributions to the health care system, will realize the importance of utilizing this process to accomplish their goals.

COMPUTERIZATION OF STRATEGIC PLANNING

It is easy to understand that cost has kept many businesses, as well as health care organizations, from being more involved in strategic planning. However, as more organizations install computer systems, the cost of obtaining data and information to do long-range planning will decrease.

Peat, Marwick, Mitchell and Company[11] recently developed a computer program to assist hospitals in their strategic planning efforts in a rapidly changing marketplace. The software program called COMPASS, was first implemented in the 726-bed Allegheny General Hospital, in Pittsburgh. Allegheny General Hospital obtained marketplace information from the American Hospital Supply Company's data base STRAPCOE. As more health care institutions acquire increased computer capability, and as improved technology drives prices down, more hospitals will have access to this form of sophisticated strategic planning.

TRUSTEE STRATEGIC PLANNING RETREATS

Hospitals have increasingly adopted the format of trustee retreats to provide an appropriate forum for developing strategic plans and long-term goals for the organization. Many administrators believe that retreats offer board members the opportunity to get away, concentrate on the major health care issues, become educated on the issues, and socialize with one another and the administrative team.[12] The retreats vary from 2- to 3-day weekends off the campus to half-day conferences on-site.

The most important goal of a trustee–administrative retreat includes identifying the institution's basic beliefs and fundamental values. It is essential that these beliefs and values be very clear and commonly agreed upon by members of the governing body and the administrative team. Without consensus on the institution's mission at the highest level, any goals or objectives for the organization would be a mere paper exercise.

The specific rationale for using a trustee retreat to develop, revise, and/or review the organization's strategic plans includes the following:

- To provide a distraction-free, relaxed environment to educate the board on health care market issues.
- To build an atmosphere of unity and confidence in the future.
- To educate the board on new responsibilities and challenges.
- To develop trust and a working rapport between the board and the administative team of the hospital.
- To establish realistic and appropriate goals for the organization and to develop a "common vision" for the hospital to which everyone is committed.

FORECASTING ALTERNATIVE FUTURE SCENARIOS

A minority of hospitals have separate planning departments and/or professional planners to develop their strategic plans. This trend is changing, however. Hospitals are realizing the importance of assessing driving trends in the past and present for the purpose of planning business strategies for future survival. The new discipline of health care futurism is devoted to forecasting future trends and demands for health care services based on assessment of current trends utilizing various forecasting techniques.[9] Futurists work to identify the "zone of feasible forecasting" which is somewhere between the perfect future forecast and no forecast at all.

There are both quantitative and qualitative forecasting techniques that are used to determine future alternatives available in the health care industry. Quantitative techniques are discussed in detail in Chapter 7. The most frequently used qualitative forecasting technique in health care is the scenario. A *scenario* is a combination of projections, assumptions, and forecasts of current trends into a story of potential future alternatives. The new discipline of futures research scans the environment for driving trends that could be indicators of the future, and then develops these alternative future scenarios.

It is believed that the future is not a matter of chance but rather a matter of choice. This choice is enhanced by the forecasting of potential scenarios and the selection of the desired future. This process includes these steps:

1. Identify the organization's present situation.

2. Identify the organization's strengths and weaknesses.
3. Identify the driving trends in the environment that could be threats and opportunities for the organization.
4. Construct possible alternative future scenarios based on the driving trends.
5. Identify the desired future for the organization.
6. Develop a plan of action to actualize the desired future.
7. Implement the plan.
8. Evaluate and implement contingency plans as needed.

Coile[9] identified four socioeconomic scenarios that are used by the Health Network of America Futures Program for developing scenarios for their member hospitals. Table 6-5 outlines these four health care scenarios, which are analogous to the common socioeconomic scenarios.

The four potential scenarios outlined for the health care industry can be classified by the probability of their occurrence in the following manner:

1. Status quo scenario
2. Least likely, least preferred scenario
3. Most likely, most preferred scenario
4. "Wild card" scenario, or possible, but not likely, scenario

Figure 6-4 shows a probability model of scenario alternatives for a given environment or data base situtation.

Using this model, Coile has identified the probabilities of the four scenarios for the health care institution:

1. Status quo scenario—High technology, computerized hospital
2. Least likely, least preferred scenario—national health system with an increase in chronic care

---

Table 6-5   Alternative Future Scenarios

Socioeconomic Scenarios	*Health Care Scenarios*
1. Coming boom 2. Competition 3. Decline and stagnation 4. Voluntary simplicity	High technology Conglomerates National health system Wellness

(Coile RC Jr: Managing tomorrow's health care organizations. Lutheran Hospital Society of Southern California, 1983)

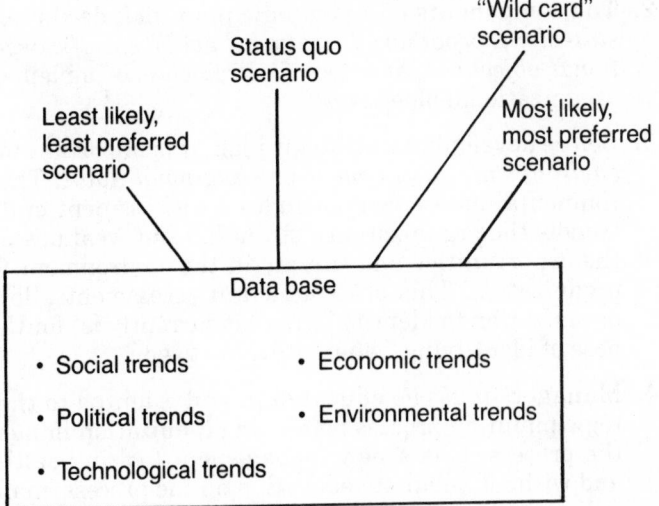

Figure 6-4. *Probabilities of alternative scenarios. (Thanks to Russell Coile for outling this model during an informal meeting.)*

3. Most likely, most preferred scenario—conglomerates of multi-hospital for-profit and non-for-profit chains

4. Wild card scenario—wellness resulting from an increase in personal responsibility for health; a decrease in the need for acute care services

In summary, scenario development is not a sure-fire method for predicting the future. However, if an organization truly believes it has the capacity to choose their future, it can be assisted in attaining the desired future by identifying current driving trends in the environment and developing strategic plans to accomplish that desired future.

SUMMARY

The major concepts that the nurse manager/administrator needs to understand from this chapter on strategic planning, include the following:

1. *Strategic planning* is long-range planning that extends 3 to 5 years into future. *Operational* or *annual planning* is short-term and determines the yearly goals of the organization. *Medium-range planning* is the planning for programs that extends from 1 to 3 years, or the length of time it requires to develop a program or new service.

2. The components of a strategic plan include the *mission statement, broad organizational goals, specific organizational objectives,* and *specific strategies* to implement the organizational objectives.

3. Before developing a strategic plan, it is important to do an *environmental assessment* or *situational audit.* The environmental assessment includes an assessment of driving trends, the organization's strengths and weaknesses, and the opportunities and threats in the environment for the organization. This environmental assessment allows the organization to identify "where it currently is" for the purpose of identifying "where it wants to go."

4. Managers must be educated in and oriented to the strategic planning process before an organization implements the process. It is a new management tool in health care, and without adaquate education on the process, managers will resist the process.

5. Goal setting and planning are crucial in the rapidly changing health care setting. If organizations and managers fail to plan, they can plan to fail. A strategic plan is also vital to assist an organization in evaluating how well it is doing in attaining its goals.The strategic plan allows the organization to focus all its valuable resources in the direction of its predetermined goals.

6. *Scenario development* is writing potential stories about future alternatives for the organization. After the alternative futures are identified, the organization can choose its desired future and allocate resources in the direction of the desired future. The use of scenario building for an organization's strategic plan acknowledges that the future is a matter of choice, rather than chance. If the organization does not plan, its future is a matter of chance.

7. Using a brainstorming process, a *WOTS-up analysis* identifies the organization's weaknesses, opportunities, threats, and strengths. By looking very closely at these aspects of the organization, it is possible to set more realistic, attainable goals.

8. The process of strategic planning can be used for health care organizations, professional organizations, and individual career planning. It is basically a form of long-term goal setting that is a critical component for the success of any group or individual.

REFERENCES

1. Goldsmith J: The health care market: Can hospitals survive? Harvard Business Rev 52:103, 1980
2. Domanico L: Strategic Planning: Vital For Hospital Long-Range Development. Hospital and Health Services Administration, Summer 1981
3. Steiner G: Strategic Planning, p 4. New York, Free Press, 1979
4. Thompson, Strickland: Strategy and Policy: Concepts and Cases, p 7. Business Publications, Inc., 1981
5. Koontz H, O'Donnell C: Essentials of Management, p 160. New York, McGraw-Hill, 1978
6. Camillus J: The practice of strategic planning. New York, The National League for Nursing Publication, No. 21-1803
7. Overcoming strategic planning obstacles. Hospitals, December, 16, 1982
8. Drucker P: Management: Tasks, Responsibilities, and Practices. New York, Harper & Row, 1974
9. Coile RC Jr: Managing Tomorrow's Health Care Organizations. Lutheran Hospital Society of Southern California, 1983
10. Overcoming strategic planning obstacles. Hospitals, December 16, 1982
11. Kuntz E: New program promises hospitals better tools for strategic planning. Modern Healthcare, p 52, January 18, 1985
12. Yanish D: Retreats offer forum to discuss strategic plans, long term goals. Modern Healthcare, p 31. January 18, 1985

ADDITIONAL READINGS

1. Anthony RN: Planning and Control Systems: A Framework for Analysis. Boston, Harvard Business School, 1965
2. Camillus JC: Evaluating the benefits of formal planning systems. Long Range Planning, June 1975
3. Cetron M, O'Toole T: Encounters with the Future: A Forecast of Life into the 21st Century. New York, McGraw-Hill, 1983
4. Guth WD: Formulating organizational objectives and strategy: A systematic approach.JBusiness Policy, Fall 1971
5. McMillan N: Planning for Survival. Chicago, The American Hospital Association, 1978
6. Schlenker R: The future of the health care organization. Health Care Management Review, Spring 1980

Quantitative Methods for Decision Making

HEALTH CARE MANAGERS are being expected to make high-quality decisions more quickly because of a rapidly changing environment. Therefore, managers can benefit from any techniques that can assist them to make better decisions. This chapter outlines the fundamentals of decision analysis and describes a number of quantitative decision methods that could be used by nurse managers and/or administrators to help them make better decisions on a day-to-day basis.

There are entire books written on quantitative decision-making methods. This chapter will focus on defining only a few quantitative decision-making methods and associated terminology. In addition to defining specific terminology, the chapter will actually walk the reader through the steps for some of the methods that can be used by the nurse manager/administrator on a daily basis. The focus of this chapter is to familarize the reader with the terminology, scope, and purpose of quantitative methods, and to explain the actual process of a few methods that could be useful in a health care management environment.

OBJECTIVES

After completing this chapter, the reader will be able to

1. Define basic terminology for decision-making methods.
2. Develop a GANTT chart for a program or project.
3. Develop a PERT chart for a program.
4. Do a cost–benefit analysis to identify the costs and benefits for a particular alternative.
5. Identify the purpose of using quantitative methods in decision making.
6. Outline four quantitative methods that are useful for decision making in a health care setting.
7. Calculate the expected times for a network model by using the weighted-average equation.
8. Outline the critical path of a network model.
9. Diagram a shortest-route network problem and apply the methodology to a nursing management situation.
10. Calculate projected monthly patient days by the moving-averages method.
11. Calculate projected annual patient day volumes using the least-squares method.
12. Explain the difference between the least-squares method and multiple-regression forecasting techniques.
13. Develop a decision-tree analysis for a nursing management decision.

MANAGEMENT RESPONSIBILITY FOR PROBLEM SOLVING

The basic responsibility and function of a manager is to solve problems. The basic process of problem solving follows these nine steps:

1. Assess the environment.
2. Define the problem.
3. Identify possible solutions.
4. Analyze the solutions.
5. Choose the best solution.
6. Implement the best solution.
7. Evaluate the solution.
8. Revise the solution.
9. Assess the environment.

These steps can be arranged to form a model for a manager's responsibility for problem solving. A model is a fundamental concept in quantitative analysis and was briefly explained in Chapter 1. A *model* is a representation of the real world or a real problem. By constructing a model, one can reduce a problem to its most significant components and understand it more easily. The steps in the managerial problem-solving model can be diagrammed as shown in Figure 7-1.

PURPOSE OF QUANTITATIVE METHODS

Quantitative methods focus mainly on step 4 of the model, or the analysis of the possible solutions. There are two methods for analyzing alternatives in problem solving: quantitative and qualitative.[1] *Qualitative analysis* utilizes the manager's judgment, past experience, intuition, and expertise to identify the most appropriate solution to the problem. Execution of this method of analysis improves with experience. It is very appropriate to use this form of analysis in many problem situations, and its usefulness and effectiveness should not be minimized.

Quantitative analysis, on the other hand, converts various alternatives into quantitative or numerical terms. By converting complex alternatives into similar numerical terms, the strengths and weaknesses of each alternative can be identified more easily. Analyzing various alternatives for solving prob-

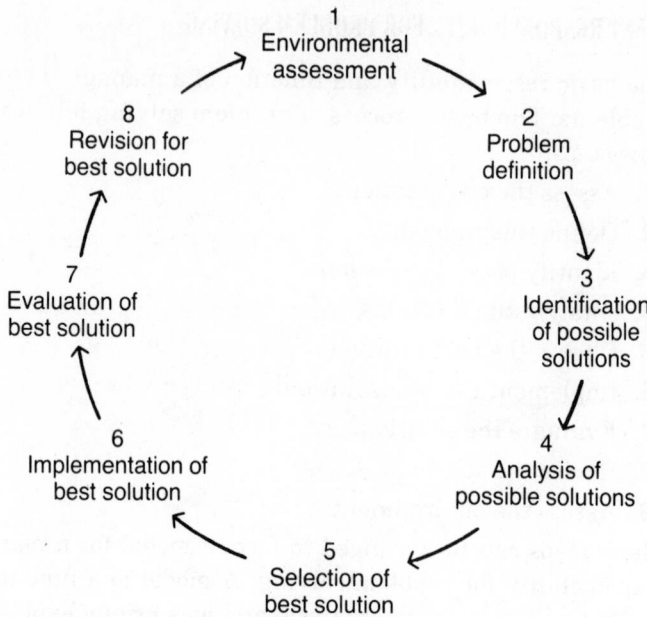

Figure 7-1.   *Managerial problem-solving model.*

lems by using a combination of qualitative and quantitative methods is the most effective method for choosing the best alternative in decision making.

For example, if a nursing administrator is interviewing three different individuals for a department director position, it would be a very effective strategy to rate each candidate numerically on predetermined criteria. When analyzing the interview data, the numbers may be very similar for all three candidates because of their qualifications. The administrator, however, might not "feel right" about the most highly rated individual. Therefore, it would be important for the administrator to take into account both the somewhat "objective" (although no assessment can really be objective) quantitative numerical ratings, as well as the "gut level" assessment or qualitative data. The "best" decision may not be to choose the individual with the highest number of points. The quantitative ranking of each candidate, however, assists the administrator in focusing on specific priorities and allows ranking of each candidate's ability in those areas. It is important, again, to stress that the manager makes the decisions and is accountable for those decisions. Qualitative and quantitative methods are merely tools to help the decision-maker evaluate the alternatives to make the best decision.

BASIC MODEL OF A PROBLEM

Most management problems in health care today are very complex, and will continue to be so in the future. However, they can all be simplified by putting them in terms of the basic problem model (Fig. 7-2).

It is easy to see from this model that all problem situations are made up of three basic major components:

1. Present condition or situation
2. Alternative paths
3. Goal situation

After creating a model for a complex situation, the manager can easily identify the information and/or data he or she needs to understand a complex issue in order to make a decision.

There are various kinds of models that managers can use. An *iconic model* is a concrete model, such as a physical model of a new contruction project.[1] It is usually done on a much smaller scale than the real-life object because of cost and practicality. An iconic model allows the manager to actually see that nothing is left to chance. A *symbolic* or *abstract model* is a model that uses diagrams and/or numbers to represent an actual thing. Quantitative methods are examples of symbolic models. Other examples of iconic and symbolic models are displayed in Table 7-1.

VALUES

Human values are an integral part of the problem-solving process and need to be mentioned in a chapter on decision making.[2]

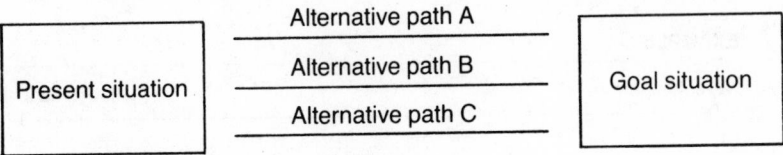

Figure 7-2. *Basic problem model.*

Table 7-1   Qualitative and Quantitative Models

Iconic Models	Symbolic Models
Model airplane	Profit and loss statement
Construction model	Balance sheet
Doll house	Blue prints
Wax molds	Pert chart
	Gantt chart

Individuals assess their present state or environment based on their value system. They identify their future goals based on what they value and what they do not value. Finally, they identify and select alternative solutions or paths to obtain their goals based on their value system. Values are one reason that one manager chooses one alternative and another chooses a different alternative, given they have identical present and goal states.

PROBABILITY THEORY

As previously mentioned, decision making for health care managers is becoming more complex on a daily basis. One of the reasons for the increase in complexity is the uncertainty of the environment. Uncertainty of future events increases the challenge of decision making for managers. In the 19th century, Simon (1749–1827) combined the ideas of early scientists to develop the first general theory of probability, which was developed to deal with the uncertainty in decision making.[1]

Probability theory identifies the chance that something will happen. Probabilities are expressed in percentages (*e.g.,* 50% chance), as fractions (*e.g,* 1/2), or as decimals (*e.g.,* .5). When expressed as a decimal or fraction, probabilities range from 0 to 1. A *0* probability means that something will never happen, whereas a probability of *1* means that the event will always happen.

EXAMPLE

Never happen		Always happen
0--	5--	1

When percentages are used to identify probabilities, 0%

means an event will never happen, and 100% means it will always happen.

EXAMPLE

Never happen   Always happen

0%--50%--100%

An *event* is defined as one or more possible outcomes that can occur. For example, when a head nurse schedules an employee to work on a day there are two possible events that can occur.

Event 1: The employee can show up for work.

Event 2: The employee can call in sick.

When the head nurse schedules a specific number of staff for a weekend, he or she includes a mental note of the probability that someone will call in sick.

There are three methods to identify or measure probability for specific events[1]:

1. The *classic method* of calculating probability:

$$\frac{\text{Number of times an event occurs}}{\text{Total number of different events}}$$

If the head nurse identifies that historically one staff member has called in sick each shift on the weekend, and there are usually six staff members scheduled on each shift, he or she could calculate the probability of someone calling in sick for each shift in this manner:

SAMPLE CALCULATIONS

$$\text{Probability of a sick call} = \frac{\text{number of sick calls}}{\text{total number of sick calls and number of staff reporting for work}}$$

$$P = 1/6$$

$$P = .17, \text{ or } 17\%$$

There is a 17% chance that someone will call in sick. When the head nurse has this information he or she can decide if additional staff need to be scheduled to ensure that an adequate number of staff is available to care for patients.

2. The *relative frequency method* of determining probability calculates the number of times an event occurred over a longer period of time, based on historical data.

   If the same head nurse counted 40 sick calls on the weekends for an entire month, the probability of sick calls can be calculated in this manner:

SAMPLE CALCULATIONS

---

6 Staff scheduled/shift $\times$ 6 weekend shifts $\times$ 4 weekends = 144 events

$$P = \frac{40 \text{ sick calls}}{144 \text{ total possible events}}$$

$$P = 40/144 = .27 = 27\%$$

There is a 27% chance of a sick call on the weekend. The head nurse can use this information to decide whether to schedule additional staff to adequately care for patients. Given a 27% probability that someone will call in sick the head nurse definitely should identify a back-up plan for adequate staffing on the weekends.

3. The final method for identifying probabilities is the *subjective* or *intuitive method*. This method is used when there are no mathematical data available to calculate probabilities. The assignment of probabilities by the subjective method may use limited evidence or just good quessing. For example, imagine that Christmas Eve and Christmas Day fall on a weekend, and that the head nurse needs to calculate the probability of sick calls for the unit on this holiday weekend. She has already calculated the probability for weekend sick calls to be 27% by the relative frequency method but believes that because the weekend is also a holiday, the probability of sick calls will be greater. The head nurse may not have any data from the previous year regarding sick calls on Christmas. Therefore, she assigns a subjective probability of 40% to sick calls because she feels that there will be a greater frequency of sick calls because of the combination of a holiday and the weekend.

SAMPLE CALCULATIONS

$$\text{Probability of sick calls} = \frac{\text{number of sick calls}}{\text{total events}}$$

$$40\% = \frac{\text{number of sick calls}}{6 \text{ staff} \times 6 \text{ shifts} = 36}$$

$$40\% = X/36$$
$$36 \times .40 = X$$
$$14 = X, \text{ or number of sick calls}$$

Given that the head nurse believes the probability for sick calls on this holiday weekend to be 40%, there could be a total of 14 sick calls for the six holiday shifts. The head nurse decides to staff one extra person each shift to compensate for the 14 possible sick calls. (In this situation, traditionally there has been no decrease in census on this unit on the weekend or holidays.)

Rules of Probability

The probabilities that have been discussed so far involve the probability of mutually exclusive events. *Mutually exclusive events* deal with either/or situations. Either the employee comes to work or calls in sick. One event does not affect the occurrence of the other, and therefore the events are mutually exclusive. When events are mutually exclusive, the sum of the events must equal the total events, and the probabilities for each event must total 1, or 100%.

SAMPLE CALCULATIONS

Number of sick calls + number of staff who came to work = total number of staff scheduled
$$14 + 22 = 36$$

Probability of sick calls + probability of staff coming into work = 1.0, or 100%
$$.4 + .6 = 1.0$$
$$40\% + 60\% = 100\%$$

This probability rule can be more easily written like this[3]:

$$P(A \text{ or } B) = P(A) + P(B)$$
where: A = number of sick calls
B = number of employees that work
P = probability that something will happen

CASE EXAMPLE

A nursing administrator wants to decrease turnover in the nursing department. She gathers the following historical data for terminations for the past 5 years, based on years of nursing experience.

Years of Experience	Number of Terminations
0–1	45
1–3	20
3–5	10
>5	6
Total	81

The administrator can use this data to calculate the probabilities for turnover for nurses with different numbers of years of experience. By calculating these probabilities, the nursing administrator can make better hiring decisions to decrease turnover rates and orientation costs.

Sample Calculations

Event	Years of Experience	Terminations	Probabilities
A	0–1	45	45/81 = 55%
B	1–3	20	20/81 = 26%
C	3–5	10	10/81 = 12%
D	>5	6	6/81 = 7%

P(A) + P(B) + P(C) + P(D) = 100%
55% + 26% + 12% + 7% = 100%

This example shows that there is a greater probability (55%) for nurses with less than 1 year of experience to terminate within the first year of employment, as compared with nurses having more than 5 years of experience (7%). By doing such a probability analysis of historical termination data, the nurse administrator can make more effective hiring decisions in the future to decrease turnover in the nursing department. By decreasing employee turnover, the administrator can decrease the cost of orientation time and reduce labor costs.

INVENTORY MANAGEMENT

Inventory management has become more important in acute care institutions. In an environment of strict cost containment and efficiency, the costs associated with maintaining inventory becomes an issue for all managers. Nursing has traditionally stock-piled or "hidden" extra supplies on the unit so that they would "never run out." Keeping large amounts of cash tied up in inventory makes a significant impact on the hospital's cash flow. Besides the fact that large inventories tie up cash, there are additional factors of inventory management that add to the organization's costs.

There are specific costs associated with maintaining inventory that can be minimized. These costs include the following[1]:

1. *Ordering costs* are the costs associated with placing an order. Ordering costs cover the cost of processing a purchase order, receiving goods and putting them in inventory, cost of stationery, and the salaries of all individuals handling the order.

2. *Carrying costs* are the costs that result from maintaining an inventory, such as storage space costs, record keeping, interest lost from money invested in inventory, taxes, spoilage, and obsolescence. When items in inventory (*e.g.,* food) spoil or become obsolete or outdated, the organization must write-off those costs as a loss.

3. *Stockout costs* are the costs an institution experiences as a result of being out of an item. If a patient must be transferred to another facility as a result of a stockout, the institution experiences a loss in patient revenue.

The hospital must consider the lead time of a commodity for deciding when to reorder. If the lead time is not taken into account, the hospital may run out before the shipment is received. Running out of stock is called a *stockout*. Stockouts are especially undesirable in an acute care setting, where lack of a particular item could cause patient discomfort or even death. Stockouts can cause an increase in health care costs if patient care is delayed for a period of time or patients must be transferred to other facilities to obtain the necessary equipment or supplies.

Safety stock refers to the amount of stock that is maintained above normal stock levels to avoid a stockout. The *reorder point* is the level of stock that signals the reordering of a particular item. The reorder point is determined by multiplying the average daily use by the lead time and then adding the safety stock.

EXAMPLE[1]

Reorder point = (average daily use × lead time) + safety stock

---

If a head nurse wants to determine the inventory level and reorder point for admit kits on the unit, he or she could calculate those levels in the following manner:

SAMPLE CALCULATIONS

- Step 1. Identify the average number of admissions on the unit = 10
- Step 2. Identify the lead time for ordering the admit kits = 1 day
- Step 3. Identify the level of safety stock of admit kits = 4 kits

     Reorder point = average daily use × lead time + safety stock
     Reorder point = 10 × 1 + 4
     Reorder point = 14

By performing these calculations, the head nurse knows that he or she needs to reorder admit kits when the floor stock is down to 14 kits so the unit does not run out. It is important to understand that if admissions increase or decrease markedly, he or she would need to recalculate the stock levels.

Management's goal is always to minimize the cost of maintaining inventories without running out of key items. This can be accomplished by minimizing ordering costs, carrying costs, and the costs associated with stockouts.

LINEAR PROGRAMMING

Linear programming is a quantitative methodology to determine the best use of an organization's resources. A linear programming solution describes the best combination of two or more variables to maximize an organization's resources or minimize its costs.[4] A maximization linear programming problem seeks to determine the best combination of two or more variables that maximize organizational revenue or outcomes. Sample problems in a health care institution follow:

SAMPLE PROBLEMS

Maximization

Identify the combination of medical beds and psychiatric beds for Hospital X that would maximize revenue.

Minimization

Identify the staffing mix of RNs and LVNs for an intermediate care unit that meet minimum standards of care and minimize cost per unit of service.

The maximization or minimization equation is called the *objective function*. The objective functions of these two examples can be written as follows:

SAMPLE OBJECTIVE FUNCTION

Maximize daily profit = profit/day for med-surg bed × no. of med-surg beds
+ profit/day for psychiatric bed × no. of psychiatric beds

Max. profit = $250 × no. med-surg beds + $150
× no. of psychiatric beds

$Max._p$ = $250 (x) × $150 (y)

where $Max._p$ = maximize daily profits
x = med-surg beds (no. of)
y = psychiatric beds (no. of)

Minimize costs = RN cost $\times$ no. of RNs + LVN cost $\times$ no. of LVNs
Min. costs = \$112 $\times$ no. of RNs + \$64 $\times$ no. of LVNs
$\text{Min.}_c = \$112(x) + \$64(y)$
where: Min._c = minimize costs
x = no. of RNs
y = no. of LVNs

The next important component of a linear program is the constraints. A *constraint* is a limitatation expressed as a mathematical inequality. Referring to the maximization example, two contraints are identified.

CONSTRAINTS

1. The number of psychiatric beds must be at least 30 more than the number of med–surg beds, or

$$y \geq x + 30$$

2. The total number of beds is not to exceed 200 beds, or

$$x + y \leq 200$$

The linear maximization problem for hospital beds is summarized as follows:

SAMPLE CALCULATIONS

Objective function

$$\text{Max.}_p = \$250(x) + \$150(y)$$

Constraints

$$y \geq x + 30$$
$$x + y \leq 200$$

In order to solve for x and y, we must first eliminate the inequalities in the constraints. This is done by simply changing the inequalities to equalities like this:

CONSTRAINTS

$$y \geq x + 30 \text{ becomes } y = x + 30$$
$$x + y \geq 200 \text{ becomes } x + y = 200$$

The next step is to get the unknown quantities on the same

side of the equation, so that we can solve for them. Whenever a function is performed on one side of an equation, the same function must be performed on the other side of the equation.

In the first constraint, or $y = x + 30$, we want to put both unknowns on one side of the equation, and the value on the other side. We want to move the x from the right side of the equation to the left side. We can do this by subtracting (x) from both sides of the equation:

$$y - x = 30$$

We do not need to revise the second equation, because it is already in the proper format, or:

$$x + y = 200$$

The next step is to solve for these two equations simultaneously by adding them together:

CALCULATIONS

$$\begin{array}{r} y - x = 30 \\ \underline{y + x = 200} \\ 2y + 0 = 230 \\ y = 115 \end{array}$$

We can solve for x by substituting 115 for y:

$$\begin{array}{r} x + y = 200 \\ x + 115 = 200 \\ x = 200 - 115 \\ x = 85 \end{array}$$

After solving for x and y, the objective function or maximization for profit can be solved:

CALCULATIONS

$$\begin{aligned} \text{Max.}_p &= \$250(x) + \$150(y) \\ \text{Max.}_p &= \$250(85) + \$150(115) \\ \text{Max.}_p &= \$21{,}250 + \$17{,}250 \\ \text{Max.}_p &= \$38{,}500 \end{aligned}$$

This linear program problem has identified that if a hospital wants to maximize its daily profits, makes $250 profit on each medical–surgical bed and $150 on each psychiatric bed, and has these constraints:

1. Must have at least 30 more psychiatric beds than medical–surgical beds.
2. Can have a total of only 200 beds.

The best combination of beds is

- 115 Psychiatric beds, and
- 85 Medical–surgical beds

The next linear program problem to be solved is the minimization problem. The head nurse of an intermediate care unit wants to calculate the staffing mix of RNs and LVNs to use for a shift that minimizes the salary cost per patient or unit of service, while meeting certain constraints. (Staffing patterns in this unit are the same for all three shifts.) The objective function or minimization equation is written like this:

$$\text{Minimize cost} = \frac{\$112(\text{no. of RNs}) + \$64(\text{no. of LVNs}) \times 3 \text{ shifts}}{\text{Average patient census}}$$

$$\text{Min.}_c = \frac{\$112(x) + \$64(y)(3)}{25}$$

Constraints

1. With an average daily census of 25 patients, the unit must have a minimum of five direct caregivers per shift.

$$\text{No. of RNs} + \text{no. of LVNs} \geq 5$$
$$x + y \geq 5$$

2. In the intermediate care unit, there must be twice as many RNs as LVNs, because of the patient acuity.

$$\text{No. of RNs} \geq 2 \times \text{no. of LVNs}$$
$$x \geq 2y$$

Just as with the maximization problem, the first step in solving for x and y is to make equalities out of the inequalities.

$$x + y \geq 5 \text{ becomes } x + y = 5$$
$$x \geq 2y \text{ becomes } x = 2y$$

The next step is to rearrange the equations, so that they may be added together:

$$
\begin{array}{llll}
x + y = 5 & \text{remains } x + y = 5 \text{ remains} & x + y = 5 \\
x = 2y & \text{becomes } x - 2y = 0 \times (-1) = & -x + 2y = 0 \\
\hline
& & 0 + 3y = 5
\end{array}
$$

$$
\begin{aligned}
3y &= 5 \\
y &= 1.7 \\
\text{if } y &= 1.7 \\
x + y &= 5 \\
x + 1.7 &= 5 \\
x &= 5 - 1.7 \\
x &= 3.3
\end{aligned}
$$

Because it is not possible to staff with a fraction of a nurse, the head nurse would interpret these results as follows:

$$
\begin{aligned}
x &= 3.3 \text{ changed to 4 RNs} \\
y &= 1.7 \text{ changed to 2 LVNs}
\end{aligned}
$$

To calculate the minimization cost, the numbers are substituted for the unknowns:

SAMPLE CALCULATIONS

$$
\text{Min.}_c = \frac{\$112(x) + \$64(y)(3)}{25}
$$

$$
\text{Min.}_c = \frac{\$112(4) + \$64(2)(3)}{25}
$$

$$
\text{Min.}_c = \$448 + \$128/25(3)
$$
$$
\text{Min.}_c = \$576/25(3)
$$
$$
\text{Min.}_c = \$23.04 \times 3 = \$69.12
$$

The salary cost per patient or per unit of service in the intermediate care unit is $69.12, when there are 4 RNs and 2 LVNs staffed on each shift for 25 patients. This is the lowest salary cost per patient day the head nurse can attain and meet the constraints that were identified for the unit.

GANTT CHARTS

One of the early scientific management pioneers in the century was Henry L. Gantt.[1] Gantt focused on a method to develop, plan for, and track the various phases or steps in completing a particular project. Contributions like Gantt's were the beginning of the discipline called operations research. Operations research is currently called quantitative methods or management science.

Gantt's contribution to operations research was the Gantt chart, a very useful tool for planning and managing special projects in a business setting. This tool can be used very easily and productively by nurse managers for special projects or programs for which they are responsible.

The *Gantt chart* is a project- or program-scheduling technique that outlines the work and time relationships of steps to meet a specific goal. The activities or steps that need to be accomplished are identified on the vertical axis of the chart and the timeframes are located along the horizontal axis.

Figure 7-3 shows a Gantt chart developed by a nursing administrator for the planning and implementation of an image enhancement program.

Gantt charts can be very simple or very detailed. Figures 7-4 and 7-5 exhibit various formats for Gantt charts that show various levels of detail. They are very easy to construct and allow the manager to visually see all the steps or activities that ...ust happen for the goal to be reached. This feature makes the Gantt chart an excellent planning tool for identifying the exact steps that need to be accomplished and when they need to be completed.

The Gantt chart is also a good mechanism to measure or evaluate if a project is on schedule, behind schedule, or ahead of schedule. Human nature tends to encourage the practice of procrastination, but setting deadlines promotes action to accomplish a goal.

The final strength of a Gantt chart comes from the formal recording of the goal and outlining the steps to accomplish the goal and the deadlines for goal attainment. When an individual takes the time to develop a Gantt chart, the process of writing the plan down improves the chances of goal attainment because there is a greater commitment to the goal. Individuals have many creative ideas and goals they plan to do "someday." However, when goals are written down, they have an increased chance of being achieved.

(*Text continues on p. 255.*)

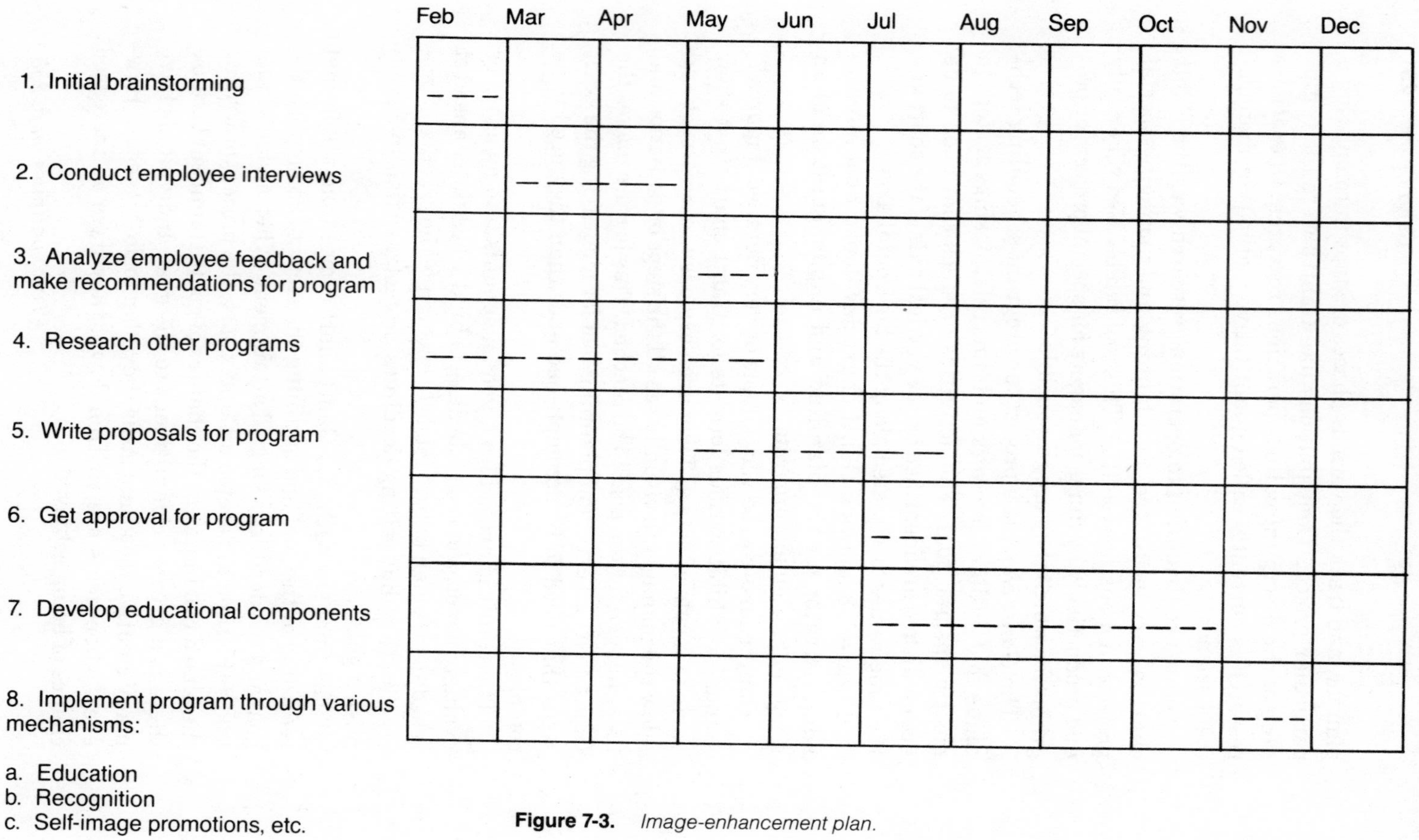

Figure 7-3. *Image-enhancement plan.*

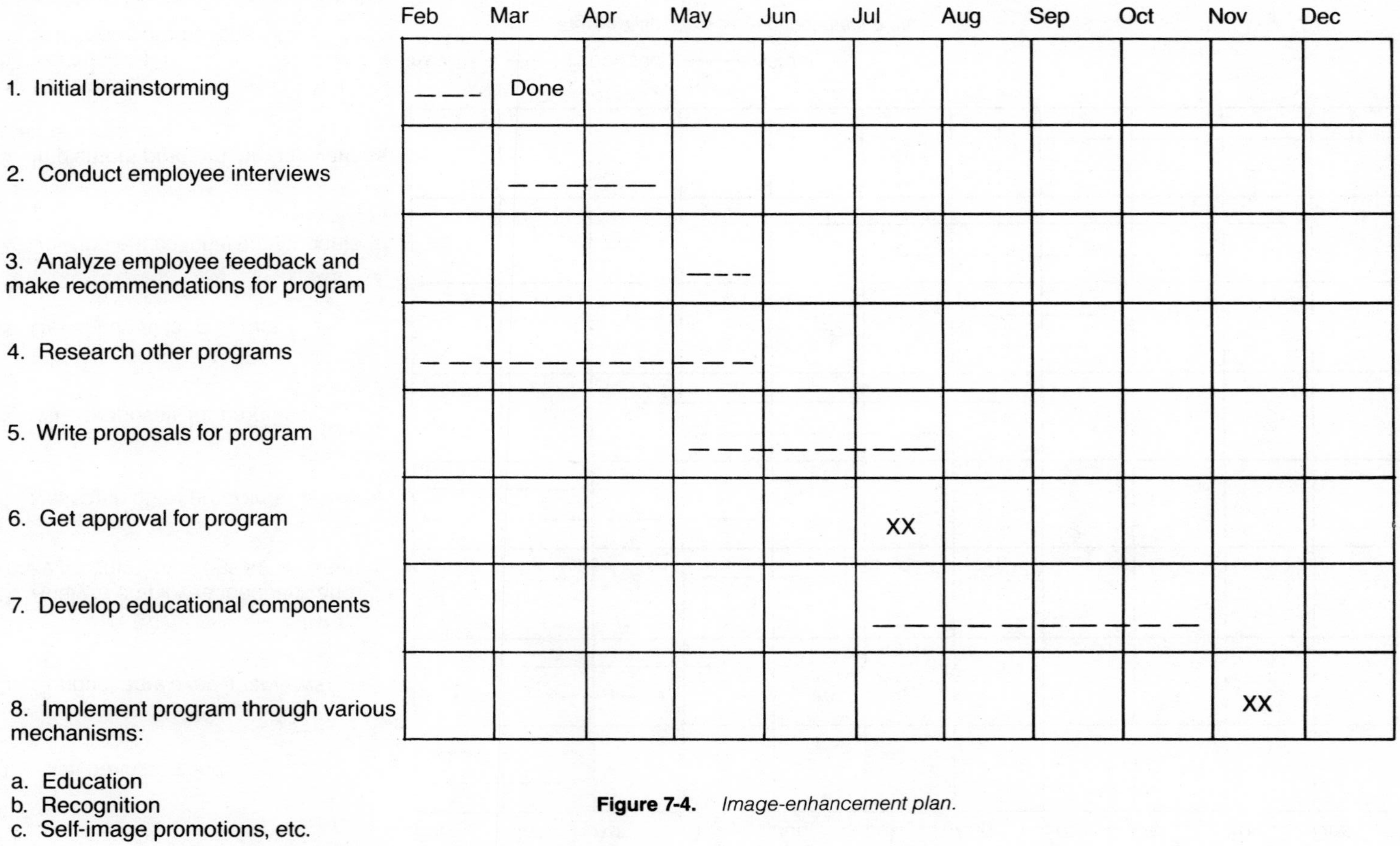

	Feb	Mar	Apr	May	Jun	Jul	Aug	Sep	Oct	Nov	Dec
1. Initial brainstorming	– – –	Done									
2. Conduct employee interviews		– – –	– – –								
3. Analyze employee feedback and make recommendations for program				– – –							
4. Research other programs		– – –	– – –	– – –							
5. Write proposals for program				– – –	– – –	– – –					
6. Get approval for program						XX					
7. Develop educational components						– – –	– – –	– – –	– – –		
8. Implement program through various mechanisms:										XX	

a. Education
b. Recognition
c. Self-image promotions, etc.

Figure 7-4. *Image-enhancement plan.*

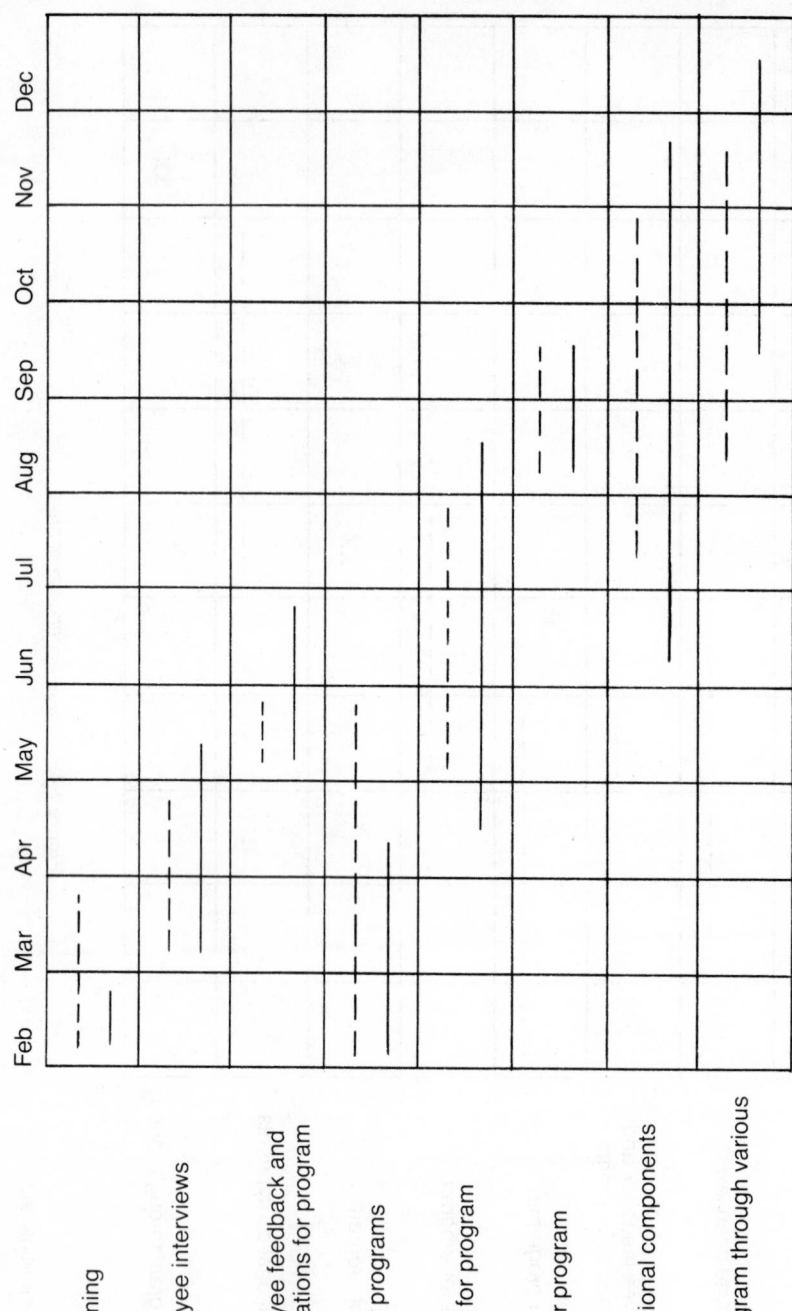

Figure 7-5. Image-enhancement plan.

Key: - - - - Proposed   ——— Actual

PERT CHARTS

Network models are graphic tools to display the relationships between activities and events to attain a specific program or project goal. Probably the most commonly used network model is the PERT chart. The *PERT* or *program evaluation and review technique* was developed in the 1950s by the Navy Special Projects Office in cooperation with Booz, Allen, and Hamilton, a management consulting firm.[1] The technique was developed specifically to keep track of the hundreds of thousands of individual tasks in the Polaris project, which included 250 contractors and over 9000 subcontractors.

The PERT technique is a somewhat more complex technique than a Gantt chart and seeks to accomplish the following objectives:

1. Identify the ending date or deadline for a project.
2. Identify each individual event and activity required to meet the goal.
3. Establish optimistic, pessimistic, and most likely time requirements for each activity.
4. Identify the predecessor events for each activity.
5. Identify the *critical path* to obtain the goal.

Before proceeding on to the actual development of a PERT chart, it is important to define some of the terms critical to PERT.

- *Activities* describe the action steps between individual events. A is the activity in this example.

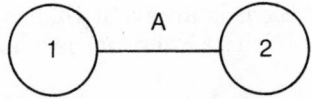

- *Events* are the completion points of activities or action steps in the network. Numbers 1 and 2 are events.

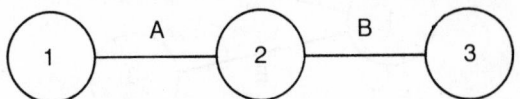

- *Float* is the amount of extra time or leeway included in an activity. If there is float time included in an activity, the activity could potentially be done in a shorter period of time.

- A *predecessor* is an event that must precede or go before other events. *Immediate Predecessors* are the specific events that must come before a particular event. Event #1 is the immediate predecessor for event #2. Event #1 is a predecessor of event #3.

- A *goal* is the primary objective of the project that is outlined in a PERT chart. It always appears as the last event. The first event is always the start or "where you are now." Event #1 is the start event and event #3 is the goal.

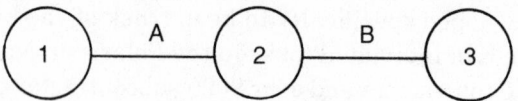

- *Critical path* is the longest path from the start to the finish or goal attainment on the PERT chart.

- A *milestone* is a particular event along the PERT network that allows the manager to evaluate progress toward goal attainment. Milestones are major critical events.[5]

- A *merge event* is an event that has two or more immediate predecessor activities that are constraining it. Event #3 is a merge event for activities A and B.

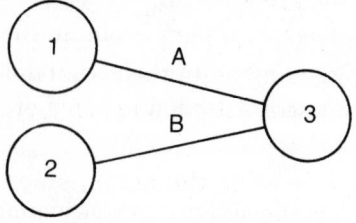

- A *burst event* is an event that is a predecessor for two or more activities.[6] Event #1 is a burst event for activities A and B.

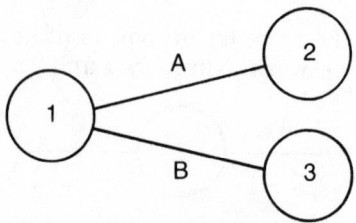

- A *dummy activity* is an activity that requires no time but must be acknowledged before another activity can occur. Activity C is a dummy activity.

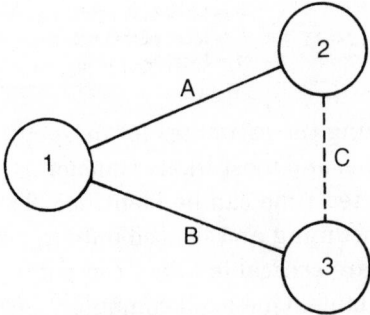

Activity A and B must be completed before event 3 or the goal can be achieved. Therefore, a dummy activity is inserted to connect the network and show the relationship of all the activities.

- *Expected time* is the time that is required to complete an activity or action step. Depending on the project and critical nature of time, approximate times can be assigned to various activities based on past experience with similar activities. Times are written on the opposite side of the activity letter like this:

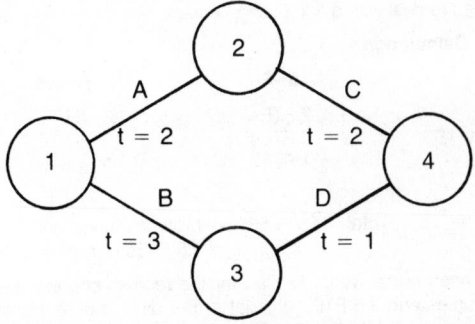

The time estimated to complete activity A is 2 weeks, activity B is 3 weeks, and so on. If accurate times are more important for the project, there is a simple equation that can be used to calculate more accurate times for PERT. This equation uses the weighted average of the most optimistic, most pessimistic, and most likely times to calculate the expected time[1]:

WEIGHTED-AVERAGE EQUATION

$$t = \frac{a + 4m + b}{6}$$

where: t = Expected time

a = Most optimistic time
b = Most pessimistic time
m = Most likely time

By identifying the estimates for most optimistic time, most pessimistic time, and most likely time for each activity, a more accurate expected time can be identified. This methodology is fairly time consuming and is used only in projects whose time determinants are critical or when computer support for calculations is available. One such computer software program for calculating times for PERT is available in a workbook entitled *Computer Models for Management Science,* by Erickson and Hall.[7] A sample expected time application follows:

CASE EXAMPLE

A head nurse is overseeing an expansion construction project on his unit. The construction project is to be completed by June 1, with patients to be admitted to the new 10-bed expansion by June 10. The head nurse wants to develop a PERT chart to assist in the planning of the recruitment and orientation of new staff for the 10-bed addition. He determines that he will need two additional LVNs on each shift, with relief to care for 10 additional patients. He decides to hire 50% full-time equivalents and 50% per diem employees to deal with a fluctuating census.

Sample Calculations

	M-F	Relief	Total
Days	2 FTEs	.8 FTE	2.8 FTEs
Evenings	2 FTEs	.8 FTE	2.8 FTEs
Nights	1 FTE	.4 FTE	1.4 FTEs
Total			7.0 FTEs

Total FTEs $\times$ 50% = full-time employees
$7.0 \times .5$ = 3.5 FTEs regular employees

The head nurse wants to plan for the recruitment and orientation of 3.5 FTEs of regular nurses and 3.5 FTEs of relief or per diem nurses. He outlines the activities he needs to accomplish before the 10-bed addition opens on June 10.

Outline of Activities

Activity/Symbol	Activity Description	Immediate Predecessors
A	Develop classified ad	none
B	Run ad in local newspapers	A
C	Post ad inhouse	none
D	Screen responses and inquiries from applicants	B, C
E	Dummy activity	none
F	Interview qualified applicants	D
G	Develop orientation program	F
H	Select qualified applicants and schedule	F
I	Dummy activity	none
J	Orient new employees	G,H
K	Open new addition	J

After identifying the activities that need to be accomplished, the head nurse must identify the most optimistic, most pessimistic, and most likely times to accomplish these activities to determine the expected time. The expected time is important because the construction is to be completed by June 1 and the unit needs to be opened by June 10, to maximize the hospital's revenue stream. The estimates for these activities will determine how soon the head nurse needs to start activity A to meet his June 10 deadline. This can be calculated by completing a table like that below by using this equation:

$$t = \frac{a + 4m + b}{6}$$

Expected Time Calculations

Activity	a	m	b	t
A	1	2	3	2
B	1	3	5	3
C	1	1	2	1.2
D	1	2	4	2.2
E		Dummy		
F	1	2	3	2
G	2	3	6	3.3
H	1	1	3	1.3
I		Dummy		
J	2	3	6	3.3
K	1	1	2	1.2

Factors that the head nurse considered in identifying most pessimistic, most likely, and most optimistic times included the following:

1. He might receive many responses from the ad right away (most optimistic), or he might receive no response for a long time (most pessimistic).
2. He might have experienced applicants who require little orientation (most optimistic), or he might have inexperienced applicants who need a great deal of orientation (most pessimistic).
3. The inservice instructor may be able to develop the orientation program right away (most optimistic), or the instructor may be backed up with other work (most pessimistic).
4. It may take a long time to schedule and interview all the qualified candidates (most pessimistic), or it might be easy to schedule and conduct interviews over a short period of time (most optimistic).

After the expected times are calculated (see table above) they can be added to the PERT diagram for the purpose of identifying the *critical path*, the longest path on the PERT chart from the start to the end, or goal attainment. In Figure 7-6, the critical path is outlined by a dotted line and represents the longest time required from the start to the end.

The major importance of the critical path lies in the fact that it represents the longest time it will take from the beginning to end of the project. Time is critical from the standpoint of completion, as well as cost. The major cost involved when identifying the time a project takes is the cost of labor. The health care industry is very labor intensive, and this is one of the causes of the high cost of providing health care services.

When seeking to reduce expenses or the cost of a project, one

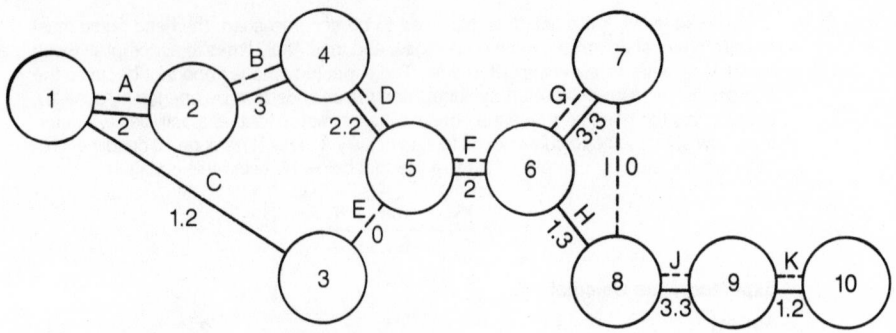

Figure 7-6. *PERT chart and critical path.*

must consider reducing the amount of time it takes to complete the project. When a PERT chart has been diagrammed and the critical path identified, the cost of the project may be reduced if the project is completed in a shorter period of time. However, if more human resources are needed to "crash" or reduce the critical path, the cost of the project may actually increase. The *crash cost* is the cost associated with completing a project on a crash basis to reduce its completion time or critical path.[1]

The cost of each activity can also be placed on the PERT chart to determine which activity to crash. Remember that in some instances, crashing an activity can decrease costs. However, when some activities are crashed, the cost of the project increases because of factors such as overtime and so on.

This has been a somewhat simplified overview of PERT but one that should enable any nurse manager to use the technique for management projects. It is believed that any detail beyond what was discussed here has limited usefulness for the nurse manager on an ongoing basis. The focus of this chapter is on a level of detail and sophistication that is useful without being overwhelming or beyond practical use.

SHORTEST ROUTE NETWORK

Another network model that could be useful for nursing is the shortest Route Network Model. In the *shortest route model,* the manager is trying to find the shortest distance from a beginning to a destination (end).

This model would be very useful for a director of a home

health agency who wants to identify the shortest, most efficient way for the home health nurses to schedule their home visits.

CASE EXAMPLE

A home health director expects each home health nurse to report to the hospital at 7 AM to receive assignments and pick up supplies, charts, and so on. The agency pays the nurses 20¢ per mile for their visits, and consequently the director wants to identify the shortest, most efficient route for the nurses to travel to their home health visits to minimize travel expenses.

The director diagrams the shortest route model in Figure 7-7; to show the distances involved between the hospital, the patients' homes, and the individual nurse's home. (The nurse does not have to return to the hospital at the end of the day.)

After diagramming this model, the director can outline the shortest route for the home health nurse to travel to make his or her home health visits. The home health nurse can be given a copy of the model with the assignment. The director can use the model and calculations to keep track of the mileage the home health nurse submits for reimbursement on a monthly basis.

The shortest route is calculated by adding up the totals of each potential route and selecting the shortest distance.

FORECASTING TECHNIQUES

At one time or another, every nursing manager is expected to forecast future trends for patient census and labor and supply requirements. Therefore, it is very beneficial for nurse managers to understand how to perform various forecasting techniques to increase their accuracy in determining future demands for services and departmental needs.

There are both qualitative and quantitative forecasting techniques.

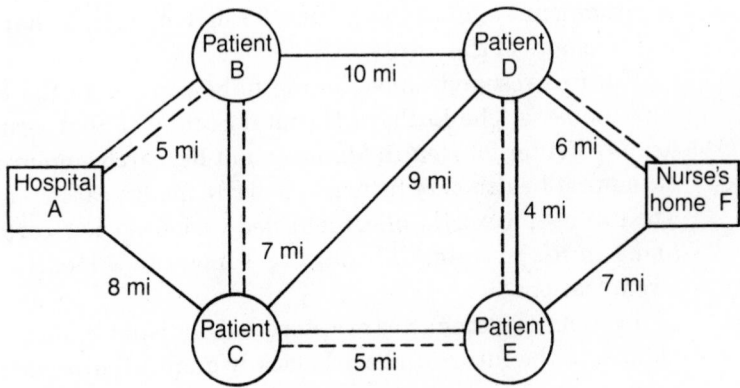

Figure 7-7. *Shortest route model for home health visits.*

Qualitative Forecasting Techniques

Qualitative forecasting techniques use subjective data from the past and present to identify future trends. The Delphi method and scenario development are two examples of qualitative forecasting techniques.

DELPHI METHOD

The *Delphi method* is accomplished when a panel of experts is interrogated by means of a sequence of questionnaires. The answers to the initial questionnaire are used to develop the second questionnaire; the responses to the second questionnaire are used to develop the third questionnaire; and so on. The final result of the Delphi method is an expert consensus decision or vision about future issues and trends. The accuracy of this forecasting method in the short and long run (2 years and more) is considered fair to very good.[1]

SCENARIO DEVELOPMENT

The second major qualitative forecasting methodology is scenario development. Scenarios use past and present trends and future assumptions and projections to develop potential future scenarios or stories about what could possibly happen.

The relatively new descipline called futures research acknowledges the necessity of identifying possible futures for the purpose of selecting the desired one. After an organization chooses a desired future, it develops and implements a strategic plan to attain that desired future. The discipline scans the environment on an ongoing basis for driving trends that could be indicators of the future.

Futures research is beginning to be popular in the health care industry. The Luthern Hospital Society of Southern California's Center for Health Management Research employed one of the first health care futurists to write health care scenarios. The futurist, Russell Coile, identified various health care scenarios in his article, "Managing Tomorrow's Health Care Organization."[8]

In summary, scenarios are stories about what could possibly happen in the future and are basically qualitative or judgmental in nature.

Quantitative Forecasting Techniques

A second kind of forecasting methodology is quantitative in nature. The quantitative forecasting methods that will be discussed include moving averages, least squares method, and regression analysis. *Quantitative forecasting methods* project future demand or volume in numerical terms, based on historical trends or causal relationships.

WEIGHTED MOVING AVERAGE

The *weighted moving average* technique is a time-series method of projecting future volume. Each projected number in a moving average sequence is a weighted average of a number of past consecutive numbers. The equation used in moving averages to determine a forecast for the next month or year is as follows[1]:

MOVING AVERAGES EQUATION

$$\text{Forecast or } F = \frac{3M^1 + 2M^2 + M^3}{6}$$

where: F = forecast
M^1 = latest month's information
M^2 = information from 2 months ago
M^3 = information from 3 months ago

If a head nurse wants to project future patient days for the purpose of developing the budget, the weighted moving average method would be accomplished as shown in Table 7-2.

Table 7-2 shows projected patient days for April, May, and June by the weighted moving average method to be 611.5, 603.6, and 610.8, respectively. The actual patient days experi-

---

Table 7-2   Weighted Moving Average Calculation of Monthly Patient Days

Month	*Actual Patient Days*	*3-Month Weighed Moving Average Forecasting*
Jan	630	
Feb	612	
Mar	605	
Apr	600	$((3 \times 605) + (2 \times 612) + 630)/6 = 611.5$
May	620	$((3 \times 600) + (2 \times 605) + 612)/6 = 603.6$
Jun	612	$((3 \times 620) + (2 \times 600) + 605)/6 = 610.8$

Table 7-3 Comparison of Weighted Moving Averages and Actual Figures

	Forecasted	Actual
Apr	611.5	600
May	603.6	620
Jun	610.8	612

enced were 600, 620, and 612, respectively. The weighted moving average method projects the next month's patient days based on the fluctuations actually experienced over the past 3 months. This method allows the administrator to project short-term future volume measures that are more sensitive to current trends than are annual budget projections. Table 7-3 compares the forecasted patient days calculated by the weighted moving averages method with the actual patient days.

This forecasting method allows the manager to update projections of patient days after actual figures are identified to make the next month's projection more sensitive to the actual patient days most recently experienced. The patient day projections that a hospital uses for budget purposes are not as sensitive to monthly trends as are the projections calculated by the weighted moving average method.

LEAST SQUARES METHOD

The next time-series method of forecasting is the least squares method of calculating trends. This method is more appropriate for determining annual patient day trends.

CASE EXAMPLE

A nursing administrator has gathered 5 years of past data for the purpose of projecting future patient day volumes.

Year	Actual Patient Days
1981	29,800
1982	30,800
1983	33,100
1984	34,280
1985	35,000

The least squares method of projecting future volume involves the solving of three algebraic equations.[1] The first equation for fitting the straight line trend for patient days is written like this:

$$\hat{Y} = a + bX$$

where: Y = the dependent variable or projected patient days
a = the point at which the trend line crosses the y axis
b = the rate of change or slope of the line (patient day growth per year)
X = the independent variable of time

The second equation is for calculating b, or the slope of the line:

$$b = \frac{\Sigma XY - n\overline{XY}}{\Sigma X^2 - n\overline{X}^2}$$

where: b = slope of the best-fitting line
Σ = the sum of a number of values
X = values of the independent variable or time
Y = values of the dependent variable or patient days
$\overline{X}$ = the mean of the values of the independent variable of time
$\overline{Y}$ = the mean of the values of the dependent variable of patient days
n = number of data points involved (5 in our example)

The mean of a group of numbers is the average. An independent variable is a value that is not dependent on another variable or number. A dependent variable or number is affected by another variable or number.

The third equation determines the y intercept, or a:

$$a = \overline{Y} - b\overline{X}$$

where: Y = the mean of the values of the dependent variable of patient days
a = the Y intercept
b = the slope of the line
$\overline{X}$ = the mean of the independent variable of time

These three equations can be solved by setting up a table like Table 7-4. The first column represents the point on the graph. The second column represents the independent variable of time, or X. The third column represents the dependent vari-

Table 7-4

Data Point	Year (X)	Patient Days (Y)	(X)(Y)	X²
1	0-1981	29,800	0	0
2	1-1982	30,800	30,800	1
3	2-1983	33,100	66,200	4
4	3-1984	34,280	102,840	9
5	4-1985	35,000	140,000	16
Totals	$\Sigma X = 10$	$\Sigma Y = 162{,}980$	$\Sigma XY = 339{,}840$	$\Sigma X^2 = 30$

$$\bar{X} = \Sigma X/5 \qquad \bar{Y} = \Sigma Y/n$$
$$= 10/5 \qquad\quad = 162{,}980/5$$
$$= 2 \qquad\qquad = 32{,}596$$

able of patient days, or Y. The fourth column represents the multiplication of patient days (X) by the year (Y). The fifth column represents the year, or (x), squared. (A number is squared by multiplying it by itself; for example, $2^2 = 2 \times 2 = 4$.)

The calculations in Table 7-4 are completed for the following unknowns:

$$\Sigma X \qquad \bar{X}$$
$$\Sigma Y \qquad \bar{Y}$$
$$\Sigma XY \qquad \Sigma X^2$$

Then it is possible to solve the equations for the unknowns a and b.

SAMPLE CALCULATIONS

$$b = \frac{\Sigma XY - n\bar{X}\bar{Y}}{\Sigma X^2 - n\bar{X}^2}$$

$$= \frac{339{,}840 - (5)(2)(32{,}596)}{30 - (5)(4)}$$

$$= \frac{339{,}840 - 325{,}960}{10}$$

$$= \frac{13{,}880}{10}$$

$$b = 1{,}388$$

$$a = \bar{Y} - b\bar{X}$$
$$= 32{,}596 - (1{,}388)(2)$$
$$= 32{,}596 - 2{,}776$$
$$a = 29{,}820$$

After solving the equations for a and b, the nursing administrator can calculate projected patient days (Y) for 1986 by inserting 5 in place of the X in the equation (1981 is 0; therefore, 1986 is 5) and inserting the actual numbers for a (29,820) and b (1,388).

SAMPLE CALCULATIONS

$$Y = a + bX$$
$$Y = 29,820 + (1,388)(5)$$
$$= 29,820 + 6,940$$
$$= 36,760$$

Solving for Y using the least squares method, the nursing administrator has projected or forecast patient days for 1986 at 36,760. This forecast identifies the projected number of patient days that best fits on the trend line that was diagrammed in Figure 7-8. Figure 7-9 shows the projected patient days for 1986 graphed with the historical patient days from years 1981–1985.

Year	Patient days
1981	29,800
1982	30,800
1983	33,100
1984	34,280
1985	35,000
1986	36,760 (projected)

MULTIPLE REGRESSION FORECASTING

The final method of forecasting trends discussed in this chapter is the *multiple regression equation*. This method is very similar to the least squares method; however, it incorporates two independent variables rather than one.[1]

The least squares equation is

$$\hat{Y} = a + bX$$

and the multiple regression equation is

$$\hat{Y} = a + b_1X_1 + b_2X_2$$

where: a = the y intercept

b_1 = the slope of the line of the first independent variable
b_2 = the slope of the line of the second independent variable
X_1 = the first independent variable (time in years)
X_2 = the second independent variable (average length of stay for inpatients)

It is possible to use the same case as for the least squares method and add an additional variable. The first independent variable, or X, is still years, and the second independent variable is the average length of stay for patients. This method is used to calculate Y, or projected patient days for 1986.

Just as in the least squares method, there are three equations to use to solve for the unknown quantities of a, b_1, and b_2. These equations are as follows:

$$\Sigma Y = na + b_1 \Sigma X_1 + b_2 \Sigma X_2$$
$$\Sigma X_1 Y = a \Sigma X_1 + b_1 \Sigma X^2 + b_2 \Sigma X_1 X_2$$
$$\Sigma X_2 Y = a \Sigma X_2 + b_1 \Sigma X_1 X_2 + b_2 \Sigma X_2^2$$

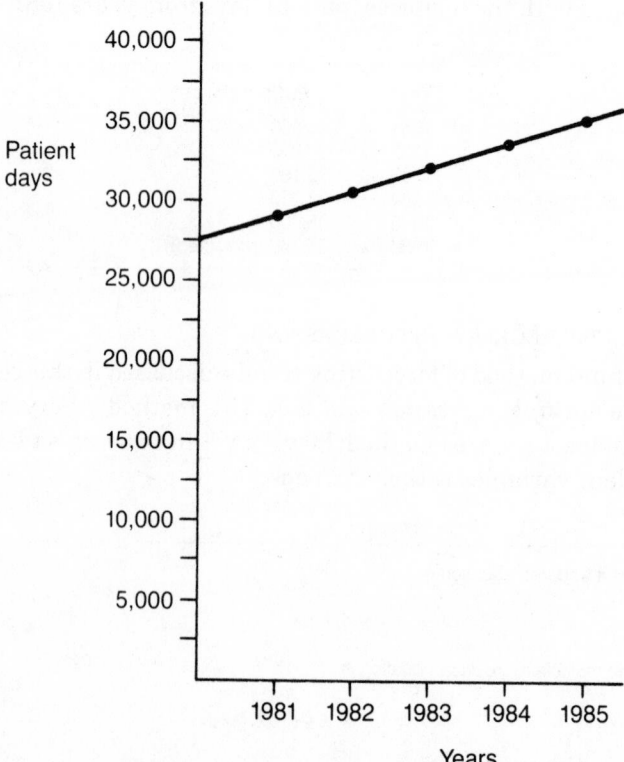

Figure 7-8.   *Trend line for patient day volume.*

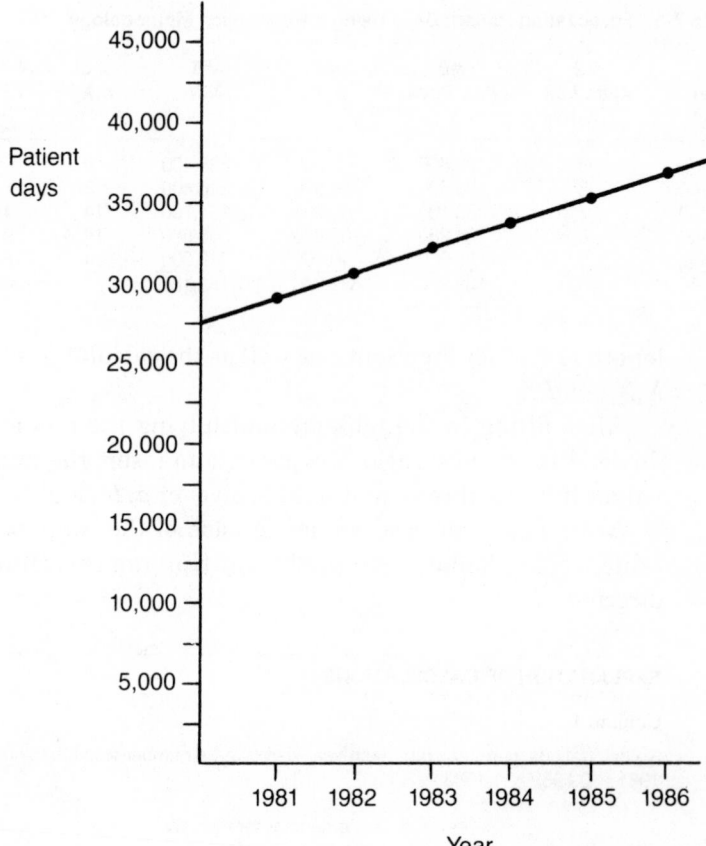

Figure 7-9. *Least squares projection of patient days graphed.*

It is important for the reader not to become overwhelmed by these equations. They are not to be memorized but looked up when a manager is solving such a projection problem. Also, as computers become more prevalent in homes and offices, these kinds of problems can be calculated using computers rather than manually. It is important for the manager to understand the rationale and basic methodology behind multiple regression analysis and be able to "walk through" a simple problem.

To simplify the calculations of this problem a table is developed, as in the least squares method. Table 7-5 shows the data and calculations inserted into the table. Table 7-5 is an expansion of Table 7-4, with the addition of the data for X_2, or average

Table 7-5   Forecasting Patient Days Using a Regression Methodology

#1 Year (X_1)	#2 Aver. Los (X_2)	#3 Pat. Days Y	#4 X_1Y	#5 X_2Y	#6 X_1X_2	#7 X_1^2	#8 X_2^2
1981(0)	8	29,800	0	238,400	0	0	64
1982(1)	8	30,800	30,800	246,400	8	1	64
1983(2)	7	33,100	66,200	231,700	14	4	49
1984(3)	6	34,280	102,840	205,680	18	9	36
1985(4)	6	35,000	140,000	210,000	24	16	36
10	35	162,980	339,840	1,132,180	64	30	249

length of stay for inpatients, as well as the calculations for X_2Y, X_1X_2, and X_2^2.

After filling in the table by multiplying the unknowns as directed in the headings, it is possible to insert the numerical values into the three equations to solve for a, b_1, and b_2.

Note: The numerical values in each of the columns of the table were calculated simply by multiplying the columns as directed.

EXPLANATION OF CALCULATIONS

Column 1

No calculations were required. Each year was given a number value, beginning with 0. 1981 = 0, 1982 = 1, 1983 = 2, etc.

$$X_1 = \text{the number for the year}$$

Column 2, or X_2

X_2 is the second independent variable, or the average length of stay for patients. These numbers were obtained from historical annual data.

Column 3, or Y

Y equals annual patient days. These numbers were obtained from actual annual data.

Column 4, or X_1Y

These figures were calculated by multiplying the number in column 1 by the number in column 3. For example,

$$0 \times 29,800 = 0$$
$$1 \times 30,800 = 30,800$$
$$2 \times 33,100 = 66,200$$
$$3 \times 34,100 = 102,840$$
$$4 \times 35,000 = 140,000$$

Column 5, or X_2Y

These figures were calculated by multiplying the numbers in column 2 (X_2) by the numbers in column 3 (Y). For example,

$$8 \times 29{,}800 = 238{,}400$$
$$8 \times 30{,}800 = 246{,}400$$
$$7 \times 33{,}100 = 231{,}700$$
$$6 \times 34{,}280 = 205{,}680$$
$$6 \times 35{,}000 = 210{,}000$$

Column 6, or $X_1 X_2$

These figures were calculated by multiplying the number in column 1 (X_1) by the numbers in column 2 (X_2). For example,

$$0 \times 8 = 0$$
$$1 \times 8 = 8$$
$$2 \times 7 = 14$$
$$3 \times 6 = 18$$
$$4 \times 6 = 24$$

Column 7, or X_1^2

These figures were calculated by squaring the numbers in column 1 (squaring means multiplying the number by itself.) For example,

$$0 \times 0 = 0$$
$$1 \times 1 = 1$$
$$2 \times 2 = 4$$
$$3 \times 3 = 9$$
$$4 \times 4 = 16$$

Column 8, or X_2^2

These figures were calculated by squaring the numbers in column 2 (X_2).

$$8 \times 8 = 64$$
$$8 \times 8 = 64$$
$$7 \times 7 = 49$$
$$6 \times 6 = 36$$
$$6 \times 6 = 36$$

Next, the numbers in each column are added up. The symbol Σ refers to the "sum of the numbers."

By plugging these figures into the equations it is possible to solve for the unknowns:

Calculations

Equation 1:
$$\Sigma Y = na + b_1 \Sigma X_1 + b_2 \Sigma X_2, \text{ or}$$
$$162{,}980 = 5(a) + b_1(10) + b_2(35)$$

Equation 2:
$$\Sigma X_1 Y = a \Sigma X_1 + b_1 \Sigma X_1^2 + b_2 \Sigma X_1 X_2$$
$$339{,}840 = a(10) + b_1(30) + b_2(64)$$

Equation 3:
$$\Sigma X_2 Y = a \Sigma X_2 + b_1 \Sigma X_1 X_2 + b_2 \Sigma X_2^2$$
$$1{,}132{,}180 = a(35) + b_1(65) + b_2(249)$$

The next step consists of solving for the unknowns, a, b_1, and b_2, by simultaneously solving the three equations. The three equations are written as follows:

#1: $\qquad 5a + 10b_1 + 35b_2 = 162{,}980$
#2: $\qquad 10a + 30b_1 + 64b_2 = 339{,}840$
#3: $\qquad 35a + 64b_1 + 249b_2 = 1{,}132{,}180$

One of the unknowns must be restated in terms of the other two unknowns so that the remaining two unknowns can be determined. It is possible to restate equation 1 to eliminate a in this manner:

#1: $5a + 10b_1 + 35b_2 = 162,980$ becomes:
                       $a = 32,596 - 2b_1 - 7b_2$

Next proceed to equation 2 and substitute the above equation for the unknown, a:

Equation 2: $10a + 30b_1 + 64b_2 = 339,840$ becomes:

$$10(32,596 - 2b_1 - 7b_2) + 30b_1 + 64b_2 = 339,840$$
$$325,960 - 20b_1 - 70b_2 + 30b_1 + 64b_2 = 339,840$$
$$325,960 + 10b_1 - 6b_2 = 339,840$$
$$10b_1 - 6b_2 = 13,880$$

Equation 3: $35a + 64b_1 + 249b_2 = 1,132,180$

$$35(32,596 - 2b_1 - 7b_2) + 64b_1 + 249b_2 = 1,132,180$$
$$1,140,860 - 70b_1 - 245b_2 + 64b_1 + 249b_2 = 1,132,180$$
$$- 6b_1 + 4b_2 = -8,680$$

After these substitutions are completed, the two unknowns can be solved for. This can be accomplished by multiplying equation 2 by 2 and equation 3 by 3 and adding the equations.

#2: $10b_1 - 6b_2 = 13,880 \times 2 = 20b_1 - 12b_2 = 27,760$
#3: $-6b_1 + 4b_2 = -8,680 \times 3 = -18b_1 + 12b_2 = -26,040$
                                               $2b_1 + 0 = 1,720$
                                               $b_1 = 860$

After the value for b_1 is determined, it is possible to solve for b_2 by substituting 860 for b_1 in any of the three equations:

Equation 2: $10b_1 - 6b_2 = 13,880$
                               $10(860) - 6b_2 = 13,880$
                               $8,600 - 6b_2 = 13,880$
                               $-6b_2 = 5,280$
                               $b_2 = -880$

Solving for a

$$a = 32,596 - 2b_1 - 7b_2$$
$$a = 32,596 - 2(860) - 7(880)$$
$$a = 37,036$$

Now that all the unknowns are calculated, it is possible to insert the original multiple regression equation to calculate projected patient days in 1986 with an average length of stay (LOS) of 5 days for inpatients. The calculated unknowns are as follows:

$a = 37,036$ $X_1 = 5$ (for 1986)
$b_1 = 860$ $X_2 = 5$ (for 1986)
$b_2 = -880$

Multiple Regression Equation

$$Y = a + b_1X_1 + b_2X_2$$
$$Y = 37,036 + 860(5) + (-880)5$$
$$Y = 37,036 + 4,300 - 4,400$$
$$Y = 36,936$$

Patient days are projected to be 36,936 in 1986. This represents a continued upward trend in patient day growth, but also a decrease in actual length of stay for patients admitted to the hospital. This regression method of forecasting allows the manager to take into account decreasing patient length of stay, as well as a general growth in volume. This method allows the manager to forecast future volume when there is more than one variable affecting future projections. This is particularly useful in the 1980s, when acute care institutions are experiencing significant decreases in length of stay.

COST–BENEFIT ANALYSIS

Cost–benefit analysis attempts to evaluate the costs and benefits of one or more alternatives for the purpose of making cost-efficient decisions. This technique has become more important in the health care industry as a result of the increased awareness of scarce resources. A cost–benefit analysis puts the alternatives in dollar terms for the purpose of deciding which alternative is the most reasonable.

It must be acknowledged here that there are many factors or attributes of different alternatives that cannot be quantified, such as quality, sturdiness, and efficiency. Therefore, when comparing alternatives by means of a simple cost–benefit analysis, some assumptions must be included. Some of those assumptions should deal with the following issues:

Assumptions to Consider When Making a Cost–Benefit Analysis

1. Quality of the product produced
2. Efficiency of the alternative
3. Potential downtime, repair costs, etc.
4. Adequacy of the alternative for the job

One simple cost–benefit analysis method compares the initial costs, annual upkeep or operational expenses, interest rates, and lifespans of the alternatives to identify the best choice. These factors are put in terms of present value so that the alternatives may be more accurately compared.[3] (Net present value was outlined in Chapter 2.)

An example of the use of cost–benefit analysis in a health setting follows:

CASE EXAMPLE

A nurse administrator is evaluating two different nurse call systems for installation in the three medical–surgical units in his hospital. The nurse call systems are similar in their capabilities, service policies, ease of repair, and availability and cost of parts. Both companies have good reputations. Alternative A costs $150,000 initially, with annual operating expenses of $8,000. Alternative B has an initial cost of $125,000, with annual operating costs of $10,000. Both systems are expected to have an economic life of 10 years. (The *economic life* is the projected period of time the system will be functional). The current interest rate is 8%. (Remember that the interest rate is also considered the opportunity cost. This means that if the cash were invested rather than being used to purchase the system, the organization would have an opportunity to make an 8% profit on that money. By making the purchase, the organization foregoes that opportunity for interest income.)

Sample Calculations

Key Points	Alternative A	Alternative B
Initial costs	$150,000	$125,000
Annual costs	$8,000	$10,000
Life = N	10	10
Interest rate = i	.08	.08

The equation to calculate the present cost or value of each decision is as follows:

$$\text{Price} = \text{initial cost} + \text{annual cost} \times \left(\begin{array}{c} \text{USPW} \\ i = .08 \\ n = 10 \end{array} \right)$$

where: USP = uniform-series present worth
i = interest
n = number of years in economic life

The uniform-series present worth (USPW) factors are obtained from standardized tables found in many finance textbooks. Table 7-6 shows a sample portion of an USPW table.

The USPW number is obtained by going down the column for the specific interest rate, or .08, to the number of years the system will last, or 10 years. The number at that intersection, or 6.710, is inserted into the cost–benefit equation:

Cost–Benefit Calculations

Alternative A:

$$P = \$150,000 + \$8,000(6.710)$$
$$= 150,000 + \$53,680$$
$$= \$203,680$$

Alternative A has a present cost of $203,680.

Alternative B:

$$P = \$125,000 + \$10,000(6.710)$$
$$= 125,000 + \$67,100$$
$$= \$192,100$$

Alternative B has a present cost of $192,100.

If all other factors are equal, the administrator would probably choose alternative B because of its lower cost.

When doing a cost–benefit analysis and putting each alternative into dollar terms, it is important to acknowledge the existence of certain constraints that are powerful yet difficult to quantify. These constraints include the following:

1. Legal constraints which include laws, policies, procedures, and individual rights.

2. Political constraints include relationships or loyalties to particular individuals or organizations that influence decision making.

3. Administrative constraints involve a lack of systems or capabilities to accomplish certain alternatives.

4. Technological constraints acknowledge that some alternatives are just not feasible from a technical standpoint.

5. Resource contraints include the organization's cash flow, financial position, credit rating, borrowing capability, etc.

6. Traditional or social constraints include what is generally accepted or not accepted. In health care, this is usually termed "community standard" or "standard in the community."

Table 7-6 Sample Portion of an USPW Table

N(Years)	.04	.05	.08	.10
1	.0962	0.952	.926	.909
2	1.886	1.859	1.783	1.736
3	2.775	2.723	2.577	2.487
4	3.630	3.546	3.3 2	3.170
5	4.452	4.329	3.993	3.791
6	5.242	5.076	4.623	4.344
7	6.002	5.786	5.206	4.868
8	6.733	6.463	5.747	5.335
9	7.435	7.108	6.247	5.759
10	8.111	7.722	6.710	6.144

(McKenna: Quantitative Methods for Public Decision Making, p 410. New York, McGraw-Hill, 1980)

DECISION TREES

Decision trees are graphic representations of various alternate decisions, with their accompanying results or outcomes and probabilities. Standard symbols are used in most decision tree diagrams. A square indicates a decision node. A round symbol indicates a state-of-nature node or the possible outcomes that could result from a decision. The lines connecting various symbols indicate alternatives.[1]

A simple decision tree could be used to assist a nursing manager in making a future career move. For example, a head nurse has been in her position for 4 years and is looking for greater responsibility, challenge, and economic rewards. There is an associate director of nursing position open at a nearby hospital, which has an excellent reputation. The head nurse enjoys her current job and has considered the promotional opportunities at her current place of employment. Those opportunities look slim, however, because the person in the associate director position is planning to stay for another 5 to 8 years and then retire. The head nurse therefore constructed the simple decision tree in Figure 7-10 to assist her in making her decision.

The two alternatives she identified in her career-planning decision were (1) staying in her current job or (2) applying for the other position.

The potential states-of-nature for the alternatives follow:

States-of-Nature for Alternative 1

A. Get promoted: There is a 30% chance or .3 probability that this will occur, and the payoff is a salary of $35,000.

B. No promotion: There is a 70% probability that this will occur, and then the head nurse would maintain her current salary of $30,000.

States-of-Nature for Alternative 2

A. Get the job: The payoff for this state is $40,000, and there is a 40% or .4 probability that this will occur.

B. Does not get the job: There is a 60% or .6 probability that this will occur. Then the head nurse would maintain her current salary of $30,000.

The head nurse should choose the decision that best fits her risk-averse or risk-prone nature. The head nurse will probably choose to apply for the new position if she is risk-prone because the pay-off is excellent. On the other hand, if she is risk-averse or risk-neutral she will most likely choose to stay in her current job.

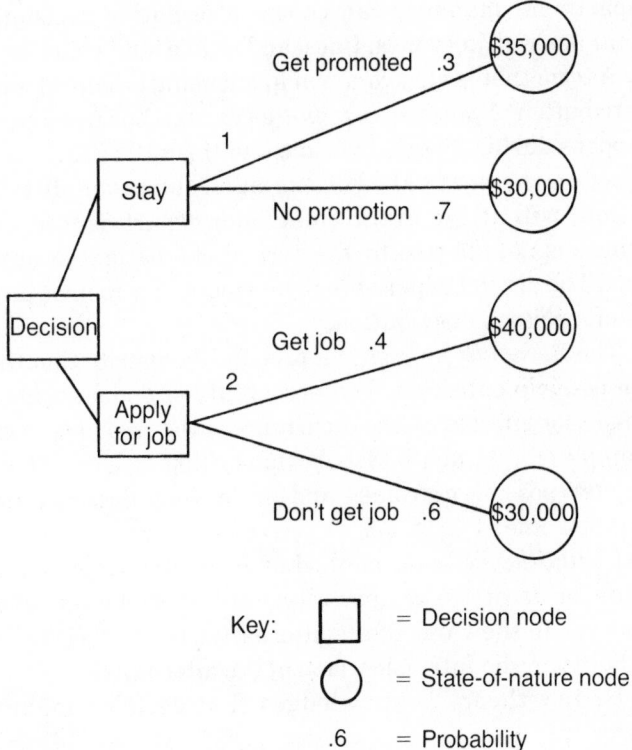

Figure 7-10. *Career-planning decision tree.*

OTHER QUANTITATIVE METHODS

There are a number of quantitative terms and methods that the nurse manager should be able to recognize in the literature but not necessarily be able to perform. A brief description of these concepts is included so that the reader has a overview of the methods.

A *queue* is a waiting line, and a *queuing model* is used to predict the consequences of various decision alternatives for a service that involves a waiting line.[3] For example, a queuing problem analysis in an emergency department would consider the rate of arrivals in the emergency department, the number of patients served per hour per physician, the service time per patient, the waiting time, and the idle time. Based on the analysis of these factors through algebraic equations, an emergency department manager can choose alternative decisions that minimize waiting times, lines, and/or idle staff time.

A term that is very common in queueing problems is poisson distribution. A *poisson distribution* exists when a call or arrival happens during a period of time and this call or arrival has no effect on the next call. For example, the probability that a patient will arrive in the emergency department at any one minute is not affected by the arrival of a patient at any other time. The arrival of patients in an emergency room is an example of a poisson distribution.

The *Bernoulli process* is a probability distribution that has two possible outcomes. The probability of one outcome occurring is not affected by the occurrence of the second outcome. An example of a Bernoulli distribution is flipping a coin. There are only two possible outcomes, and one outcome does not affect the next outcome.

Utility theory[37] is a method of assigning subjective worth, value, or utility to various alternatives. The value of utility theory is in the value of the alternative to the decision maker, rather than the intrinsic worth of the alternative.

Utility theory acknowledges that decision makers are basically

- Risk-averse (if they seek to avoid risk)
- Risk-prone (if they value risky, high-profit alternatives)
- Risk-neutral (if they are indifferent to two alternatives)

In utility theory, each alternative is assigned a utility function to evaluate its payoffs. An example of assigning utility payoffs follows:

The best payoff is assigned a utility value of 1, the worst payoff is assigned a payoff of 0, and the risk-neutral alternative is assigned a utility value of .5.

SUMMARY

This chapter has outlined various qualitative and quantitative methods and terms to assist managers in making more effective decisions. Some of the most important concepts are outlined in this summary.

1. A *model* is a representation of a real problem that allows the problem to be reduced to its most significant components and relationships for better understanding.

2. *Quantitative methods* convert alternatives into numerical terms for the purpose of analyzing the strengths and weaknesses of the various alternatives.

3. *Probability theory* identifies the chance that an event will happen or not.

$$P = \frac{\text{Number of times event occurred}}{\text{Number of total events}}$$

4. *Linear programming* is a quantitative methodology to determine the best use of an organization's resources. Linear programming problems seek to maximize benefits or minimize costs. A *constraint* in linear programming identifies the limitations of the minimization or maximization function.

5. A *Gantt chart* is a project or program scheduling technique that outlines the work and time relationships in meeting a specific goal.

6. The *PERT chart* or program evaluation and review technique is a network model that graphically displays the relationships and times between activities and events or a specific program or project. The *critical path* of a PERT chart is the path that takes the longest amount of time.

7. Estimated times to complete various activities in a network can be calculated by the *weighted average equation:*

$$t = \frac{a + 4m + b}{6}$$

8. The *shortest route network model* can be used to identify the shortest distance from a beginning node to an end node.

9. The *delphi method* is a qualitative technique for forecasting future trends that uses a panel of experts and a series of questionnaires.

10. A *scenario* is a qualitative method to forecast future trends by using past and present trends and writing a story about the future.

11. The *moving average technique* is a time-series method of projecting future volume by using a weighted average of several past consecutive numbers.

$$F = \frac{3m^1 + 2m^2 + m^3}{6}$$

12. The *least squares method* of projecting future volume solves for the slope of the line to identify future points on the trend line.

$$Y = a + bX$$
$$b = \frac{\Sigma XY - n\overline{XY}}{\Sigma X^2 - n\overline{X}^2}$$
$$a = Y - b\overline{X}$$

13. The *multiple regression method* for forecasting trends includes two independent variables and one dependent variable, and is calculated by solving the following equation:

$$Y = a + b_1X_1 + b_2X_2$$

14. A *cost–benefit analysis* converts decision alternatives into present dollar terms for the purpose of deciding which alternative is most reasonable.

$$P = \text{initial cost} + \text{annual cost} \times \left(\begin{matrix} \text{USPW} \\ i \\ n \end{matrix} \right)$$

15. A *decision tree* is a graphic representation of various alternate decisions, with their accompanying results or outcomes and probabilities.

16. A *queuing model* is used to predict the consequences of various decision alternatives for a service or situation that involves a waiting line.

17. *Utility theory* is a method of assigning subjective worth, value, or utility to various decision alternatives.

REFERENCES

1. Levin R, Kirkpatrick C, Rubin D: Quantitative Approaches to Management. New York, McGraw-Hill, 1982
2. Rubenstein M, Pfeiffer K: Concepts in Problem Solving. Englewood Cliffs, NJ, Prentice-Hall, 1980

3. McKenna C: Quantitative Methods for Public Decision Making. New York, McGraw-Hill, 1980
4. Warner D, Holloway D, Grazier K: Decision-Making and Control for Health Administration, p 193. Health Administration Press, 1984
5. Project Management, p 60. Developed by Center For Health Management Research, Lutheran Hospital Society of Southern California, 1983
6. Project Management For Health Professionals, p 64. Developed by Center For Health Management Research, Lutheran Hospital Society of Southern California, 1983
7. Erikson W, Hall O: Computer Models for Managment Science. MA, Addison-Wesley, 1983
8. Coile R: Managing Tomorrow's Health Care Organizations. Lutheran Hospital Society of Southern California, 1983

Networking Skills for Nurses

NETWORKING is not a new concept in the business world. It is a fairly new concept for nurses, however. For years, men have incorporated networking into their repertoire of business skills. They have traditionally learned the benefits of networking from their childhood involvement in team sports. Men and boys are taught from their early years to establish relationships with others who have similar interests.

Socializing or networking by participation in team sports has recently expanded to include females. As participation in softball, basketball, and soccer leagues becomes more common for grade school and high school girls, the concept of networking will also become a part of the normal socialization process for girls. Perhaps in another 10 years there will not be a need for a chapter such as this because women will have learned these concepts while growing up.

In the meantime, because 95% of all nurses are female, it is necessary to include this chapter on networking. The chapter will describe the process and implications of networking for nurses and nurse managers in a rapidly changing and competitive health care environment.

OBJECTIVES

After completing this chapter, the reader will be able to
1. Identify three methods to initiate network contacts.
2. Implement at least three networking strategies to accomplish one's career goals.
3. Implement two strategies for successful networking.
4. Identify the advantages of a mentoring relationship.
5. Identify the shortcomings of a mentor relationship.
6. Identify and implement strategies to expand one's networks.
7. Identify at least three benefits of networking.

DEFINITION OF NETWORKING

Networking is the process of creating linkages to obtain information, influence, and power. It is the process of exchanging information between strategically placed individuals who have access to ideas and other people.

Mary Scott Welch, author of the book entitled *Networking,* defines networking as "the process of developing and utilizing your contacts for information, advice, and moral support as you pursue your career."[1]

Networking is simply a fancy term for getting to know the right people and then using those contacts to assist one in accomplishing goals, solving problems, and advancing one's career. O'Connor states that networking involves "asking for help when you need it, and giving help when others need it."[2]

Fishman observes that networking has come of age in the 1980s.[3] Just as the term *relationship* was popular in the 1970s, the term *network* is popular in the jargon of the 1980s. The yippies of the 1960s have turned into the ambitious yuppies of the 1980s who seek to "leverage their personal contacts" through networking. In 1981, Jerry Rubin, an angry protester at the Democratic presidential convention of 1960, opened what he called *networking salons.* These networking salons were formal places to meet contacts and exchange business cards for future career opportunities.

Networking can be socializing with contacts about family and friends, or it can be focused on professional issues. Networking can be casual socializing and interacting with colleagues, as well as planned business meetings.

Networking requires a conscious commitment of time, energy, and resources by the professional nurse. Networking is a long-term strategy for professional and career advancement rather than a short-term strategy. The rewards of networking activity are usually not experienced in the short run. The nurse manager, therefore, must be willing to commit personal resources to networking without the expectation of reaping immediate rewards.

Persons and Wieck propose that networking's greatest benefit is in the development of both personal and professional power.[4] By establishing strong, influential network contacts, the nurse establishes a broader base of power to accomplish goals. The process of networking creates a team mentality from an individual focus. When an individual is plugged into the power of a team, the individual's power base expands.

Networking is an active process that requires a commitment of time and resources by the individual. Networking cannot be successful when accomplished by default. The manager needs to dedicate time for networking with the same discipline he or she uses to schedule meetings with subordinates or superiors. In order to make a commitment, the author advocates blocking off time on one's calendar to accomplish the following kinds of activities:

1. Make telephone calls to colleagues to "just chat" or to say "Hi." This is important even when the manager does not need anything.

2. Contact colleagues to share information on open positions, industry news, and so on.

3. Return telephone calls from colleagues and follow-up with information in a timely manner.

4. Write thank-you notes for favors received.

5. Make telephone calls to colleagues to ask for assistance with a problem. A comment such as, "I need your expertise on this problem" can be very effective.

    6. Take colleagues or potential network contacts out for lunch.

NETWORKING TO ACCOMPLISH PROFESSIONAL GOALS

The major reason for committing time and resources to networking activity is to advance one's professional career. Networking is a long-term strategy for establishing relationships, visibility, and a power base to obtain future career goals. No matter how charismatic or knowledgeable an individual is, no one can make it alone. Knowledgeable, charismatic individuals understand that their real power is obtained through their relationships and contacts with other powerful, influential people.

The first step in developing networking strategies is to identify one's career goals and aspirations. It is only after the professional nurse identifies future career goals that he or she can identify the specific networks that will be beneficial.

The steps in accomplishing career goals by networking are outlined as follows:

Action Steps

1. Identify career goals.
2. Identify existing networks.
3. Identify the appropriate networks to obtain career goals.
4. Initiate network contacts.
5. Cultivate network contacts.
6. Utilize network contacts for career advancement.

    Step 1: Identify career goals. This seems like a fairly simple issue. However, in the author's experience, it is usually a difficult task for nurses to accomplish. Nurses traditionally have a lot of different things they would like to do in the future. These ideas are many times focused in very different directions. The nurse, therefore, spends a great deal of time going in different directions, rather than concentrating all efforts and resources in the pursuit of one specific goal. Many lack the confidence or vision to make a specific commitment to a long-term professional goal.

    This could be true because in the past many women went into nursing as a part-time job until they got married or had children. They did not go into nursing for a long-term career. This trend is changing, however. Networking is a professional career strategy that requires long-term vision and commitment (at least 3–5 years).

Step 2: Identify one's existing networks. List all professional contacts and categorize them by answering the following questions:

- Are one's professional contacts influential in the arena of future career goals?
- Are network contacts diversified and from various areas of interest?
- Are contacts limited to the manager's organization, city, and state?

Step 3: When the nurse identifies future career goals, it is possible to identify specific networks and network contacts that would be beneficial to cultivate. If the nurse desires to become known and make a contribution in a specific clinical area, it is important to become active in the appropriate professional organizations.

The author will outline a specific networking case study. A critical care assistant head nurse identifies that she desires to be a director of one or more critical care units. The nurse is planning to stay within the general geographic area where she currently lives. The nurse has a diploma degree in nursing and is CCRN certified. The nurse could develop the networking plan shown in Table 8-1 to assist her in obtaining her professional goal within 3 to 5 years.

STRATEGIES FOR SUCCESSFUL NETWORKING

Strategies for successful networking are broad guidelines for the nurse manager to obtain long-term career goals in specific areas. Additional strategies to develop a broader base of network contacts and increased access to information and personal power to accomplish one's goals could include the following:

- Subscribe to a non-nursing business magazine for women. Periodicals like *Savvy* and *Working Woman* give the female nurse ideas that other successful professional women have developed in their specific fields. Nurses need to broaden their perspectives by using strategies for success that other women have already identified.
- Subscribe to at least one motivational and/or business magazine like *Success, Money, Business World,* and so on. The nurse manager can learn many things from other business disciplines.

Table 8-1   Networking Plan of Action

Action Step	Rationale
1. Obtain bachelor's and master's degree within 5 years.	These degrees will qualify the nurse to obtain her career goal. Her involvement in these programs will put her in contact with local nurse leaders in academia. Many positions are obtained through referrals from university professors.
2. Join local and national chapters of AACN.	Involvement in the local and national AACN will give the nurse many contacts in critical care nursing. The nurse can use local critical care nurse contacts to solve problems and share ideas. The local contacts can keep the nurse posted regarding open positions, etc. The involvement in the national AACN provides the nurse with role models to emulate in order to become a leader in critical care nursing.
3. Subscribe to journals in critical care nursing, such as Heart and Lung, Critical Care Nurse, etc.	By reading these journals on an ongoing basis, the nurse keeps current on issues affecting the field. The nurse should also become familiar with the leaders in critical care nursing that make contributions to the field through professional writings.
4. Identify a particular topic of interest, research the topic, and develop a presentation for the local chapter of AACN.	This step will assist the nurse to be able to talk in front of a group and be viewed as an "expert" on a specific aspect of nursing.
5. Attend the annual AACN convention. Introduce self to any and all nurse leaders who make an impression on the nurse.	This strategy allows the nurse to learn the corporate culture of AACN, establish relationships, and identify role models and behavior patterns of critical care nursing contacts.
6. Work hard in current position and establish a good "track record."	Networking is only successful in obtaining career goals if the individual is competent and dedicated. The nurse must establish a good track record as a leader, while at the same time establishing network contacts.
7. Write essays and papers for university classes that can be used on the job and/or submitted as an article for publication.	This strategy allows the nurse to "kill two birds with one stone." She is fulfilling her degree requirements and at the same time making a professional contribution.
8. Volunteer to serve as an officer of the local AACN chapter. Volunteer to work on chapter projects, programs, etc.	The nurse will acquire a reputation for being willing to work for the profession, be viewed as a leader, and have contacts and access to other critical care leaders.
9. Read the classified section of the local newspaper on a weekly basis.	This strategy allows the nurse to stay on top of the credentials and qualifications necessary for each position on the way to the nurse's ultimate career goal. It also allows her to keep track of turnover trends, problems, salaries, etc., at various hospitals.

- A handy method of developing a reference list of all network contacts is to maintain a business card file. Plastic business card files or notebooks can be purchased at any stationery store for under $10. The nurse manager should ask all colleagues or professional contacts for a business card. This request flatters the contact and results in a method of keeping track of the contact in the future. It is helpful to jot a few notes on the back of the business card to remind oneself of any significant facts or expertise of the contact.

- Investing in oneself and one's future is a key networking strategy. This strategy means that the nurse manager invests money to further academic education and/or take specific courses that provide the technical skills needed to reach future career goals. The health care industry has become increasingly competitive. Nurse managers who have top administrative goals will need to equip themselves with the appropriate credentials, degrees, and skills to be successful in the present and future health care environment. The nurse manager of the present and future will need a minimum of a master's degree and preferably a doctorate degree. As the number of master's degree prepared individuals in health care administration increases, academic credentials for the nurse manager become more important and pronounced.

- The rules of the health care game are changing so quickly, it is very important for the nurse manager to keep informed. Knowledge is power, and if one is viewed as knowledgeable and current in her area of expertise, others will want to network with her to broaden their information base. The nurse manager needs to view himself or herself as a commodity to be marketed. Marketing involves finding a need and filling it. Therefore, the nurse manager needs to develop a reputation for possessing a unique personality, insight, expertise, and/or skill that is in demand. Then the manager must "promote" that skill or expertise to attract interest from others. A network is a link to information, and the manager will be considered a valuable link only if he or she possesses information or expertise that others do not have.

- After developing a strong self-image, it is important to develop good active listening skills. Individuals are impressed and flattered by people who are good listeners. Networking involves a give-and-take process, and it is typically easier to talk than listen. It is important for the networking professional to work hard at becoming a good listener to implement this give-and-take philosophy.

- The development of good communication skills is also a

key networking skill. Professionals evaluate other individuals based on their ability to communicate their skills and expertise to others. It is not sufficient just to possess a skill or special knowledge without being able to communicate those special talents to others. There are various forms of communication that are important in networking. The ability to communicate verbally, be assertive, and be outgoing is important in making personal network contacts.

• Another verbal communication skill to develop is the ability to make formal presentations to groups of all sizes. The process of making a presentation to a group of professionals allows the nurse to make numerous network contacts in a single effort. This is also a key strategy to assist the nurse in developing a strong self-image. It articulates one's thinking and position on key professional issues and creates the image of being an "expert" for the nurse.

A few points that the author has identified through experience to develop the skill of making presentations include the following:

1. Identify a current subject or topic that "turns one on" and that the nurse can really get excited about.

2. Research the topic by doing a literature search and reading everything available on the topic.

3. Develop a presentation on the subject by preparing an outline and practicing in front of a mirror or colleague.

4. Offer to give the presentation at a local professional meeting, for a colleague's organization, etc. *Hint:* If the initial presentation is given to complete strangers, one will experience less pressure or anxiety to perform perfectly. There is greater pressure on the nurse manager if the presentation is for peers or superiors. These kinds of presentations should be done after the nurse has developed self-confidence. *Another hint:* Ask one's boss or mentor to assist in identifying opportunities to practice one's presentation skills in small settings.

5. Always include an evaluation form with the presentation handouts. Review all evaluations after the presentation and accept the feedback as constructive criticism to improve future performances. Wearing an outfit that makes the speaker feel terrific and that has received compliments in the past can make a significant contribution to the presentation.

6. Ten minutes before the presentation, relax, take deep breaths, and visualize speaking in front of the group. It is

important to visualize oneself as very confident, enthusiastic, knowledgeable, and truly enjoying the presentation.

How to Make Network Contacts

It is very difficult for many individuals to feel comfortable introducing themselves to complete strangers. This feat requires either self-confidence, a commitment to take a risk, or a commitment to overcome this fear. Anyone can overcome the fear of meeting strangers by determination and practice. After walking up to a stranger, the nurse should offer her hand in a handshake and introduce herself. After a few times it becomes more comfortable and easier to do.

Two key components of this process are a strong, confident handshake and good eye contact. People are impressed with individuals who have a confident, firm handshake and make good eye contact. They tend to remember them and feel good about the contact. Whereas people tend to feel self-conscious about introducing themselves to complete strangers, the stranger usually feels very flattered and positive about the interaction. Practice seems to be the most important strategy to eliminate the fear of meeting new people. After a few successful experiences, one realizes that it is very worthwhile to take the risk to initiate contacts and conversation with colleagues whom one does not know.

Another method of initiating network contacts is to telephone a nurse leader or colleague one admires, whether the nurse has previously met the individual or not. No matter how important a person is, he or she is never too busy or too important to object to a call that acknowledges someone's admiration. For example, a nurse calls a nurse leader she admires and says, "I've read your latest article or attended your last seminar, and am very impressed with your ideas. I'd like to ask your advice on a particular problem I'm experiencing." An action such as this will always elicit a positive response. By making this contact, the nurse manager is automatically classified as a bright person because she flattered the person she called. Individuals remember people who admire them and acknowledge their leadership abilities and qualities.

It can be just as effective to write a flattering letter to a person one admires. The author received a letter from a nurse manager who attended one of her seminars, saying, "I really enjoyed your seminar and identified with your leadership style. I would love the opportunity to work with you." The author was certainly impressed with the astute perceptions of this nurse and was very flattered by the letter. If there had been an open position at the author's hospital and this nurse applied, she would have had a real advantage over other candidates. Why? Because the nurse's loyalty and support had already been demonstrated. An assessment had already been made that this nurse was very intelligent and observant because of her perceptions of the author.

A similar strategy was actually used by a nurse whom the author did interview for a nurse manager position. The author was having a difficult time making a decision between two final candidates for a head nurse position. The author then received a beautiful card from one of the candidates thanking her for the pleasant interview and complimenting her on her leadership ability and the hospital. That did it! After the card was received, it was very clear that this candidate had a real ability and skill for spotting a great leader and a great place to work. And so the card-sending candidate got the job!

A final strategy for making network contacts is to be very visible. This means that one needs to be very involved in professional organizations, projects, and committees, and be willing to commit time and energy to socialize above and beyond work hours. Successful executives in all lines of business relate that they put it in average of 50 to 60 hours per week. They do this willingly because they love their work and have specific goals they wish to accomplish. They really enjoy what they do and show it. Therefore, if a nurse manager is unable for one reason or another to commit extended time and energy, he or she may have real difficulty establishing strong network contacts, a broad power base, and an executive level position. Executive career goals require a real love of and commitment to the profession, one that usually exceeds a 40-hour-a-week job.

Additional Networking Strategies

Just as there are specific strategies and methods that result in successful networking, there are also some things that should be avoided by the networking nurse.

It is always amazing to realize how small the health care

industry actually is. The author has practiced from the Midwest to the West Coast, and when least expecting it, bumps into a colleague from a past work experience. For this reason, it is very important never to "burn your bridges behind you," and never to alienate network contacts because one never knows when or where they will show up again.

A colleague once advised, "Always treat fellow nurses as you would like to be treated, because you can never tell when one of your peers or subordinates could end up being your boss!" Although that has never actually happened, the author has been a subordinate of a nurse manager and then become that nurse's boss.

A second defensive strategy is never to gossip. If a nurse turns networking sessions into gossip sessions, he or she will acquire a reputation for being unprofessional and untrustworthy. Once such a reputation is acquired, it is very difficult to "turn back the clock" or rid oneself of such a reputation. It is important, therefore, not to become involved in gossiping in professional situations.

Along the same lines, it is important to maintain professional confidences. If a colleague shares information and instructs one to maintain the confidentiality of the information, it is important to honor this request. Once a professional has a reputation for betraying confidential information, he or she is cut off from future information that may be of a sensitive nature. It is also very difficult to change the perception that one is "unable to maintain confidences."

Expand network contacts to include individuals other than friends. Women usually network with individuals they get along with and like. This limits their power and information base to the ideas and perceptions of individuals with whom they usually agree. By networking with individuals who have conflicting ideas or ideas that challenge one's own, the manager has access to a broader range of ideas.

By networking only with friends who have similar views, one eliminates all opposing views that may have the capability of expanding and clarifying one's thinking. Opposing views and ideas assist the professional to expand his thinking, creativity, and openness. By networking with other than friends, one can keep in touch with what the opposition or competition is doing.

Individuals can learn just as much, if not more, from the competition.

When networking with colleagues who have different views, opinions, or values, it is important never to discount the information shared. Once a nurse discounts information, advice, or ideas shared in the process of networking, he or she loses access to that source of information in the future.

For example, if a nurse manager provides a colleague with advice to solve a problem, and the colleague responds by saying, "Oh, that will never work" or "That really sounds dumb," the contact will hesitate ever to share ideas with that person again. It is important always to thank a contact for an idea and keep the criticism to oneself.

Do not be afraid to ask for something from a network contact. If one never asks for assistance, one may never benefit from his networking efforts. Individuals tend to think that people can "read their mind," and know when and how they need assistance. Not so. It is important to develop a direct, up-front, assertive style and ask for what is needed. Confident, successful people know it is not a weakness to ask for help—it's just smart.

Finally, use any and all opportunities to network. Networking opportunities may come along when one least expects them, and the professional needs to be able to take advantage of all potential opportunities.

THE MENTOR RELATIONSHIP

An additional key strategy for career advancement in the business world has been the mentor relationship. Here, again, men in the business world have been traditionally more actively involved in mentoring than women.

Mentoring is a process whereby a seasoned, successful businessman takes a young inexperienced executive "under his wing" and "shows him the ropes." Usually the experienced executive identifies some admirable traits in the young executive or even "sees himself" at an earlier age. He desires to help the younger person so "he doesn't have to learn the hard way," as he did.

The mentoring relationship may be formal or informal. The

experienced executive may actually declare his intent to mentor the younger executive, or the latter may request the experienced executive to "teach him the ropes" and help him establish a track record. More frequently, individuals relate to one another in a mentor relationship with no one ever formally agreeing to do anything. This latter arrangement has been more common in the nursing profession up to this point.

Gerald Roche, president of a management consulting firm, has done research on the topic of executive mentoring. His research showed that young executives who had mentors typically advanced faster, earned higher salaries, and had more opportunities than other executives. Men traditionally are involved in mentor relationships during their college and early career years. Women, however, identify career goals in the sixth to tenth year of their working lives, and experience mentor relationships later in their careers.[1]

Functions of a Mentor

According to Levinson, a mentor has several functions. These functions or roles include that of teacher, sponsor, host, exemplar, and counselor.[5]

Teacher: In the role of teacher, the mentor shares theories, concepts, and applications that he or she has learned in the "real world." Many nursing and health care administration programs have not kept up with all the skills required on the job. The mentor is the obvious person to teach these on-the-job skills and concepts to the young nurse or manager. When the relationship is close, the mentor identifies so strongly with the mentoree, that he or she wants to spare him the pain of some of the lessons usually learned the "hard way."

Sponsor: The function of a sponsor is to speak on behalf of the mentoree and support the individual in various ways. Introducing the person to key leaders and giving the person tips on available positions, letters of recommendations, and so on make up the major sponsoring efforts of the mentor.

Host: As a host, the mentor teaches the young nurse about the culture of the organization and the profession. The mentor explains the political realities of the organization, as well as the location of real power. The mentor informs the individual about who to trust, who to avoid, what to say, and what not to say. These aspects of organizational life are usually unique to each organization, and knowledge of them can be a significant issue for new individuals trying to establish credibility in an organization.

Exemplar: The exemplar function is basically the role model function. Young nurses and managers look to nursing leaders to set the trends, pace, expectations, and so on. The mentor role provides the young professional with the ideal role model that can survive in a particular organization. If a mentor is having some political difficulties in the organization himself or herself, this could significantly interfere with the optimal socialization of the mentoree.

Counselor: The mentor functions as a counselor in that he or she advises the young professional on matters such as career moves, strategies, and timing. The young professional should use the mentor as a resource and advisor but should not be totally dependent on the mentor. A good mentor will encourage and foster independence in the mentoree.

Benefits of Mentoring

The benefits of the mentor relationship in nursing are experienced by the individual and profession as a whole. When a skill allows the professional nurse to develop more expertise and make more significant contributions, the entire profession of nursing benefits. It is believed that by acquiring a level of expertise in the business skills outlined in this text, the nurse manager can better contribute to and advance the profession of nursing in the highly competitive and challenging health care environment of the 1980s and 1990s.

Specific benefits of the mentor relationship include the following:

- Professional career planning
- Leadership development
- Professional advancement
- Increased creativity and risk taking
- Personal satisfaction
- Professional career planning for the nurse is enhanced through the close relationship with a seasoned mentor. The mentor attempts to direct the young nurse to an appropriate career track, and assist him or her to avoid the pitfalls that the mentor has encountered. The mentor

prods the young nurse to become involved in doing the "right things at the "right time." These factors or career strategies are usually not contained in formal nursing programs and are mainly learned through experience. The mentor can assist the young professional to chart the career course that maximizes the results and rewards of the resources expended by the mentoree.

- The mentor relationship assists in the development of future leaders by the role modeling of the mentor. The nurse learns how a nurse leader should act by observing the mentor's behavior and actions. The mentor acts as a counselor to the aspiring nurse to identify what organizations and activities to become involved in to establish leadership credibility. In many cases, the mentor functions by pushing and promoting the nurse. Many times, potential leaders need a little nudge or push to get involved in activities such as submitting journal articles, making presentations to professional organizations, and running for office.

- A mentor relationship between two professionals promotes an environment of increased creativity and risk taking. Whenever two or more minds are brought together to problem solve, a "third mind" results. Napoleon Hill calls this "third mind" a master mind group.[6] This third mind is the creative combination of the two minds in a mentor relationship. A young, aspiring nurse can tolerate more risk with the assistance, guidance, and direction of a seasoned nurse manager. Opportunity and potential advancements are found more frequently in high-risk situations. The presence of a mentor can assist the young nurse to function more comfortably and successfully in a high-risk environment.

- When the mentoring process works, the profession develops more leaders, who, in turn, work to advance the whole profession. Leaders are the key to the promotion and advancement of a profession or field of study and successful mentor relationships assist in the development of such future leaders.

- Finally, participation in a mentor relationship usually yields personal satisfaction for both of the individuals involved. The mentor gets a good feeling by sharing expertise and personal experiences with the young nurse. Mature, successful professionals discover that they can experience gratification from sharing their expertise with up-and-coming nurse managers.

The mentoree gains satisfaction from feeling and knowing that someone he or she admires professionally, believes enough in the mentoree to invest time and effort in coaching. He or she learns to believe more in himself or herself as a result of the mentor's belief in the mentoree's capabilities and potential.

Problems in the Mentor Relationship

Up to this point, the positive aspects of mentoring have been described. There are, however, a few potential pitfalls or problems to be aware of when engaging in such a relationship.

If a mentor lacks self-confidence and has not attained all of his or her goals, he or she may be intimidated by the success of the mentoree. If the young mentoree becomes very successful, the mentor may sabotage the future success and/or accomplishments of the young nurse. If a professional realizes his mentor has such a problem, it is important to become independent of that mentor.

A mentor may enjoy the dependency of the young nurse and provide only enough direction to maintain that dependent relationship. In the long run, this will hold the young nurse manager back and have a negative impact on the attainment of his or her career goals. It is important for the mentoree to be aware of such a situation and make provisions to become independent of such a mentor.

It is possible that the young professional possesses more talent, creativity, and drive than the mentor. If this is the case, the mentor could actually hold the aspiring nurse back. As soon as the mentoree matches the accomplishments of the mentor, it is important to find another mentor to assist him or her to aspire to even greater accomplishments.

SUMMARY

The professional nurse can benefit by incorporating networking and mentoring skills into his or her repertoire of professional tools. Some of the major concepts presented in this chapter include the following:

1. The major goal of networking is to increase the professional's information and power base to advance his or her professional career.

2. Effective networking requires a commitment of time, money, and energy resources.

3. Networking is an effective strategy to increase personal and professional power for nurses.

4. Effective networking demands that a professional not betray confidences and/or become involved in gossiping. It is very important to contribute more to network contacts than one receives in return.

5. The mentor functions as a teacher, exemplar, counselor, sponsor, and host.

6. The benefits of the mentor relationship include career planning, leadership development, professional advancement, increased creativity and risk taking, and personal satisfaction.

REFERENCES

1. Puetz B: Networking for Nurses. An Aspen Publication, 1983
2. O'Connor A: Ingredients for successful networking. JONA December 1982
3. Fishman S: The art of networkinng. Success, July/August 1985
4. Persons CB, Wick L: Networking: A power strategy. Nurs Economics, January-February 1985
5. Levinson D: The Seasons of a Man's Life. New York, Knopf, 1978
6. Hill N: Think and Grow Rich. North Hollywood, CA, Melvin Powers, Wilshire Book Co, 1966

ADDITIONAL READINGS

1. Knebel E: Dissertation: Mentoring Among Nurse Administrators. University of Houston, Summer, 1985
2. Posner M: Executive Essentials. Avon, 1982

Power and Politics
for Nurse Leaders

IN THE PAST, professional nurses have been frustrated and disenchanted with their lack of autonomy, professional standing, and economic status.[1] Historically, nurses have also avoided opportunities to obtain power and/or political clout. The profession of nursing is now learning that power and politics are neither negative nor positive concepts. The profession is learning that power and political savvy are essential in assisting professional individuals to accomplish their goals. This chapter will attempt to dispel the common myths about the nature of power and politics and identify the advantages of obtaining these skills for the nurse manager.

Most people do not like to admit that they want additional power, and nurses are no exception. This explains why a great many people do not possess power adequate to accomplish their goals. People that do possess power, on the other hand, also go to great lengths to hide the fact.[2]

OBJECTIVES

After completing this chapter, the reader will be able to

1. Define five kinds of power and delineate the kinds of power that are most effective and appropriate for nurses to use to accomplish their goals.
2. Identify two new strategies to increase one's personal power to accomplish one's goals.
3. Differentiate between the common myths and realities of politics and power in the health care setting.
4. Use at least two strategies to make the political process work in your favor.
5. Identify the six stages of personal power through which leaders progress and how power is used in each stage.
6. Define the political or bureaucratic model.
7. Identify four unique factors of politics in the nonprofit sector.
8. Identify specific symbols of power in a health care setting.

DEFINITION OF POWER

There are many different definitions of power. Individuals define power for themselves based on their own experiences, positive and negative, with power and powerful people. *Power* is commonly defined as the ability to control, influence, or act. Power is the capacity to influence and is based on the resources available to the individual or the characteristics of the individual. Weber defines power as the "probability that one actor within a social relationship will be in a position to carry out his own will despite resistance."[3] *Authority,* on the other hand, is defined as the legitimate power granted to an individual by an organization. Authority is vested in a position. The individual has power as a result of the position he holds. *Leadership* is the relationship between two or more people in which one influences the other toward the accomplishment of a goal without the use of legitimate power.

Personal power, as defined by Hagberg, is "the extent to which one is able to link the outer capacity for action (external power) with the inner capacity for reflection (internal power)."[4] Hagberg's model for personal power stages will be outlined later in this chapter.

Organizational power is the "how to get ahead" kind of power or the ability to accomplish organizational goals through other people as well as career goals within the organizational structure. It is important to note that the fair exchange of power between a leader and subordinates elicits approval by the group. However, when a leader makes unfair demands on subordinates, he is considered oppressive and is met with social disapproval or resistance. Therefore, organizational power includes an exchange of fairness in the exercising of power by the leader in return for social approval and support by subordinates to accomplish organizational goals.[5]

Another kind of power mentioned in the literature includes Clarke's notion of executive power. According to Clarke, *executive power* is "the technique of stimulating ordinary individuals with ordinary talents to achieve extraordinary results, to excel, to reach for the stars."[6] Executive power is the use of personal persuasion and influence to positively motivate individuals to accomplish organizational and personal goals. It is this kind of power that all nurse managers need to lead the nursing department. Executive power can increase productivity, change bad employee work habits to good ones, reduce absenteeism, errors, accidents, and turnover, and meet the expanded goals of the nursing department in difficult times.

Individuals believe that powerful people have special skills, knowledge, or some other quality that is very desirable. Most people want to know or be associated with powerful people and view this association as improving their own opportunities. Individuals also believe that powerful people have dominant personalities and tend to take the lead in most situations.

Because of these assumptions, powerful people tend to receive respect, fair treatment, and consideration.[7] These results are some of the reasons that many people desire more power.

McClelland and Burnham's research findings reported that good managers desire power not for personal gain, but to influence the behavior of employees for the good of the organization.[6] The use of power is positive and appropriate when it is used by managers to meet the needs of the organization and the needs of employees.

Nurses can benefit individually and collectively by acquiring additional power as defined by the author. The author believes that by assisting nurse managers to understand the value and benefits of power to accomplish their goals, their effectiveness and chances of success will increase, and their frustrations should decrease.

KINDS OF POWER

Power, authority, influence, and control are perhaps the most pervasive concepts in organizations. Their impact and consequences are experienced by individuals at all levels of the organization. A discussion of these concepts should begin with a discussion of power and authority.

Blau defines authority as possessing the following four properties[8]:

1. Authority is vested in a position. An incumbent has authority because of his or her position regardless of one's personal characteristics.

2. Voluntary compliance by subordinates is characteristic of authority. Subordinates accept voluntarily the responsibilities conferred upon them by authority figures as long as they are not oppressive.

3. Another characteristic of authority is the suspension of subordinates' judgment in advance of a command or decision. A subordinate is committed to execute a command before it is actually issued.

4. Authority can arise only in a collective contest. This property allows the official to enforce his authority over a resistant individual or minority so long as the majority are willing to enforce the authority.

A helpful model of power, on the other hand, has been identified by French and Raven.[9] This model suggests two forms of power: delegated power and earned power. There are three types of delegated power and two types of earned power. *Delegated power* is granted to the individual by the organization as a result of his position. *Earned power* is earned by the individual as a result of his or her personal characteristics and expertise.

The three types of delegated power are coercive power, reward power, and legitimate power. The two types of earned power are expert power and referent or charismatic power.

1. *Legitimate power* is the kind of power that an organization grants an individual based on his position on the organizational chart. This power is granted the individual as a condition of his job and is also known as the authority of the position. Examples of legitimate power or authority for a head nurse job usually includes hiring, disciplinary action, and firing of unit staff.

2. *Reward power* is also a delegated power of the organization and includes the distribution of rewards. A head nurse possesses the reward power to evaluate staff, which, in turn, determines their annual merit increases. Head nurses have power and influence over staff because of their power to reward staff through the evaluation and promotion processes.

3. *Coercive power* is the exact opposite of reward power, or the ability to administer punishment or disciplinary action to employees. The head nurse role has significant power and influence over employees as a result of his or her ability to discipline and/or terminate staff members. Coercive power is only a short-term strategy for obtaining employee compliance and action, however. As previously mentioned, if the manager is not perceived as exercising power in a fair manner, subordinates will exhibit resistance and lack of support for him. They will secretly plot and long for the day when they can overthrow the manager.

These first three types of power are bestowed on the individual by the organization. They are effective only in the short run and need to be accompanied by the development of earned power by the manager, for long-term effectiveness and success.

4. *Expert power* is the power earned by an individual as a result of his expert knowledge or skills. The clinical specialist role in a hospital commands power as a result of his or her expertise in a nursing specialty and attainment of a

master's degree. Staff and nurse managers value and respect the knowledge and expertise of the clinical specialist, giving the role the power to accomplish specific goals. Expert power affords the individual power and respect through knowledge or specialized information and/or skills acquired by the individual.

5. *Referent power* is the influence an individual has over another based on respect or admiration of the individual's characteristics. Referent power is the most effective long-term strategy for influencing others because the individual willingly follows the lead of the person he respects.

Expert and referent power are the most effective forms of power for the organization, employees, and individual manager. When a nursing manager can inspire and influence staff through expert and/or referent power, the staff willingly gives their respect and support to the manager. The truly effective manager/leader does not need to rely on the formal power of coercion, legitimacy, or rewards, but influences through expertise and leadership characteristics. Table 9-1 summarizes the five kinds of power, the locus of the power, and the effectiveness of each kind of power for the nurse manager.

Power vs. Authority

As stated previously, power is defined as the ability of the individual to accomplish specific goals as a result of the individual's knowledge, expertise, skills, or characteristics. Authority, on

Table 9-1 Summary of Kinds of Power

Kind of Power	Locus of Power	Effectiveness
Legitimate power	Power of position that comes with a job	Effective in short run, but ineffective in long run
Reward power	Ability to distribute rewards, that comes with the job	Moderately effective
Coercive power	Ability to administer punishment, that comes with the job	Effective in short run
Referent power	Influence based on respect for and/or identification with another person; earned by the individual.	Most effective long-term strategy
Expert power	Power through knowledge or information, earned by the individual	Second-best long-term strategy

the other hand, is the legitimate power or the right to take action that an organization bestows on an individual as a result of his position. The organization delegates authority to the individual for the purpose of attaining the goals of the organization.

Effective managers must acquire a balance of both kinds of power to be successful. If a manager possesses only power delegated from the organization, he or she will not be able to inspire and motivate staff to do their best. Staff will do the minimum that is expected of them to minimize punishment and maximize their rewards.

If a manager does not gain the respect of his employees, resulting in referent power, or have the expertise to possess expert power, he or she will not be successful in the long term. The power granted a manager by the organization is effective in the short run but cannot effectively lead or motivate a work group in the long run.

Conversely, if a manager possesses adequate referent and/or expert power and does not have the formal sanction of the organization, he will also be unsuccessful. A good example in the health care industry occurs with the clinical specialist role on a daily basis. For example, a clinical specialist in a hospital has established credibility and respect with the nursing staff, and assesses that the standards of nursing care on a specific unit are not being met adequately. She completes an in-depth analysis of the nursing care being delivered on the unit and makes the recommendation that more staff are needed to meet the predetermined standards of care. The head nurse, however, does not believe that the additional staffing is necessary and does not implement the recommendation. The head nurse also does not possess any referent or expert power in the eyes of the staff.

In this situation, there are two ineffective people. The head nurse has the legitimate authority but no personal power, respect, or credibility. The clinical specialist has the respect and credibility of the staff but no formal authority to make any decisions. Both of these individuals are ineffective because of their narrow power base. Individual power must be balanced and contain an element of both kinds of power for a manager to be successful in the long run.

Power vs. Powerlessness

Many individuals believe that power is bad or negative because of their perception that powerful people use their power to take advantage of others. However, power is neither positive or negative in itself. It is the means by which an individual gets things done. If the "things" or individuals are bad or negative, that does not mean power is bad. Figure 9-1 shows how power is a means or enabling force to assist an individual to accomplish a goal. Power is a neutral force. When a negative or positive modifier is added to the individual or the goal, the means or concept of power remains neutral.

The opposite of having the power to accomplish a goal, is the inability to accomplish a goal because of powerlessness. Whereas many people fear "powerful" people, the author proposes that just the opposite is true. Individuals should "fear" powerless people because individuals without power need to resort to methods that are manipulative, dishonest, and illegal to accomplish their goals. This proposition can be defended by looking at methods used by criminals and deviants to accomplish their goals. When individuals lack the legitimate or earned power to attain their goals, they must resort to alternative methods that may be negative or bad. Powerless people appear to be less trustworthy than powerful people. Powerful people can be very "up front" and direct in their actions because they have confidence they can accomplish their goals.

Myths and Realities of Power

Women as a group tend to shy away from the concept of power because of the many myths about the nature of power. It is important to dispel these myths before nurses can be comfortable seeking additional power to accomplish their goals. Table

Individual ———— Power ———— Goal

Bad individual ———— Power ———— Bad goal

Good individual ———— Power ———— Good goal

Good individual ———— Power ———— Bad goal

Figure 9-1. *Power model.*

Table 9-2 Myths and Realities of Power

Myths	Realities
1. Power is a goal.	1. Power is a means to accomplish a goal.
2. Power is bad.	2. Power is neutral.
3. Powerful people are ruthless.	3. Power*less* people are ruthless.
4. Power can be given to another person.	4. Power must be earned or assumed.
5. It is bad and wrong to desire more power.	5. The acquisition of power to accomplish goals reduces stress and frustration.
6. "Watergate" resulted from a quest for power.	6. "Watergate" resulted from a feeling of powerlessness.

9-2 outlines some of the more common myths and realities concerning the concept of power.

GOALS OF POWER FOR THE NURSE LEADER

The goals for the acquisition and use of power in the health care setting are of extreme interest to all nurse managers. When discussing goals that can be accomplished by the five kinds of power, the discussion will be limited to the goals of the nurse manager in an acute care setting.

Power Goals for Nurse Managers

1. To be able to get things done.
2. To be able to implement one's ideas or visions for a nursing department.
3. To be able to obtain physician support for nursing and patient care issues.
4. To be able to provide nursing staff with the appropriate human and capital resources to care for patients.
5. To be able to provide nurses with an adequate salary.
6. To be able to make a significant contribution to one's organization and/or profession.
7. To be able to survive in a difficult world.
8. To be able to advance one's career, economic, and professional status.
9. To be able to obtain respect from one's colleagues in the health care field.

10. To avoid the frustrations of ambiguity in a competitive environment.

11. To be able to be accountable for a significant issue.

As anyone can see, these are all admirable goals and ones that would definitely contribute to the status and image of the nursing profession and the individual nurse. It is because of these sample goals and these attributes of power that all nurse managers should make a conscious decision to identify specific goals to increase their personal and organizational power, and implement strategies to obtain the necessary power and political savvy to accomplish those goals.

Stages in Personal Power for the Leader

In an attempt to help managers and individuals understand the concept of power, Janet Hagberg developed a model that describes six distinct stages of personal power for a leader.[4] Hagberg's model was developed from personal experience and observation rather than from empirical research. Despite her methodology, the model warrants explanation because it makes sense and is very practical. By understanding and recognizing these power stages, one can set goals to achieve one's highest leadership potential. Hagberg's six stages of power for leaders includes the following:

Stage One: The Dictators

Stage Two: The Seducers

Stage Three: The Great Persuaders

Stage Four: The Role Models

Stage Five: The Empowerers

Stage Six: The Sages

The basic assumptions underlying Hagberg's model are as follows[4]:

1. The stages of personal power are arranged in developmental order.

2. Each stage is different from all others.

3. One can move through the stages only in the order in which they are numbered.

4. Power is described and manifested differently at each stage.

5. Each stage of personal power has positive and negative dimensions, as well as developmental struggles within it.

6. People can be in different stages of power in different areas of their lives, at different times and with different people. However, each of us has a "home" stage that represents us more truly than others.

7. Women are more likely to identify with certain stages and men with other stages.

8. Individuals do not necessarily proceed to new stages merely with age or experience, although both are factors.

9. The most externally and organizationally oriented power stages (stages one through three) show a marked contrast to the internally oriented stages (stages four through six.)

10. These stages describe the development of individuals who live in the United States in the last half of the 20th century.

Based on these assumptions, Hagberg describes leaders in each of these power stages like this[10]:

STAGE ONE: THE DICTATORS

In stage one, managers lead by intimidation and authoritarian behavior. Managers in this stage are very insecure themselves. They feel that they must use force and/or threats to motivate people. Managers that remain in this stage for any length of time are not successful in the long run.

STAGE TWO: THE SEDUCERS

When managers progress to stage two, they become more subtle in their use of legitimate power. This subtleness can be called "manipulation" of employees in order to motivate them. In this stage, managers never seem to be on top of things and are always "playing catch up." They are trying to establish their credibility as a leader but have not quite gotten the knack of it without "using" their employees.

STAGE THREE: THE GREAT PERSUADERS

When a manager becomes willing and ready to take on additional responsibility and risks, he or she progresses to stage three. Here he has learned the rules of the game and is rewarded for decisiveness, expertise, organizational savvy, and his competitive nature. He or she leads by persuasion and the power of personality or charisma. These managers have become true "leaders" because they share their goals and/or visions with their followers. They include their employees in the decision-making and the rewards in obtaining the goal. Persuaders use strategy, teamwork, commitment, persistence, and loyalty to accomplish goals with their followers. They share their successes with their "team." Middle nurse managers in this stage can be very successful.

STAGE FOUR: THE ROLE MODELS

Stage four leaders are very concerned with doing the right thing at the right time. They are concerned with the long-term success of the organization rather than short-term goals. They lead by their integrity and develop a strong trust relationship with their followers. These leaders are more people and organizationally oriented than task or results oriented. They are confident and centered to the point that they share their power and decision making with their subordinates for their development. They do not need to make the decisions themselves and they coach others to develop their abilities in these areas. Mentors are usually found in stages three or four.

STAGE FIVE: THE EMPOWERERS

Stage five leaders are very selfless leaders mainly concerned with supporting and encouraging others. They have a vision that is greater than the individual or the organization, and their actions reflect this vision. Their main goal is to empower others, and they do so without any thought of their own power or influence. Stage five leaders have defined their purpose on a higher plane, which is to serve others rather than accomplish "things."

STAGE SIX: THE SAGES

Stage six leaders are very rare and in some respects not even considered leaders. They are what we would most nearly call "gurus" and are not really prevalent in our modern organizations, because their goals are so intangible and beyond the scope of organizational life.

In summary, these stages of power development for leaders can assist the individual in identifying where they are developmentally regarding the concept of power. After identifying where one is, one can formulate strategies to move to the next developmental step to become more powerful and effective as a leader.

DEFINITION OF POLITICS

Politics is a process that results when groups of heterogeneous individuals with different goals, interests, values, and perceptions work together in organizations toward common organizational goals. The political process emerges in any environment where individuals or special interest groups have needs and demands that cannot all be met because of limited resources.

The political process acknowledges that everyone has his or her own self-interest as a primary goal in every situation. As the number of individuals involved in a situation increases, the complexity of the political process increases because of the self-interests and goals of each individual involved.

The Political Model

The political model acknowledges that there are many players who are focusing on many diverse inter- and intra-organizational problems, as well as their own self interest.[11] Players make decisions based on their perceptions of community, organizational, professional and personal goals, rather than a consistent set of objectives. Rational choice is replaced by the pulling and hauling that is called politics. Decisions are made based on individual goals, organizational routines, the power and skill of the proponents, and the power and skill of the opponents in a specific issue.

The purpose of developing political savvy for the nurse manager is to define various ways to obtain one's goals, while identifying the other players, their goals, and the effect they will have on the manager's goal attainment. Whenever an individual has a goal while functioning in an organization, it is important to identify what others in the system also want and use that information to plan one's strategy to accomplish one's goal. When a manager identifies a strategy to obtain a goal without acknowledging the effects other players will have on the goal, the manager has not planned for the inevitable resistance and sabotage from other actors in the organization and consequently may not meet the goal.

The political process provides the organization with an ability for reaching some consensus on who in the organization receives what and when they receive it. In a participative organizational environment, the principal mechanisms for achieving these consensus decisions are through negotiation, compromise, persuasion, and bargaining. The give-and-take that occurs in the political process sometimes alters the original goals to the point that they are unrecognizable. This give-and-take process makes rational individuals sometimes arrive at seemingly irrational decisions.

One goal of politics is to control and influence the opposition. The opposition is any person or group that thinks differently. Oppenheimer (1914) identified three major components of politics[12]:

1. The presence of an authority structure to coordinate activities
2. An all-or-nothing involvement by members
3. A treatment of outsiders as adversaries or the opposition, rather than as competitors

To a certain extent, these components dictate behavior by individuals in a political environment. They are "unwritten" laws that are to be observed if one wants to be able to play the "game" of politics.

The Political "Game"

The political "game" also involves four basic concepts that are important for a "player" to understand and acknowledge to be successful in playing the game. These four basic concepts include the following[11]:

- Who are the players?
- What are the goals, interests, and stakes of each player?
- How much power does each player have?
- What are the rules and rewards in the game?

By identifying these four concepts in each political encounter, one can better assess the situation in order to make the best decision. The first important step in becoming politically savvy is to acknowledge that politics do exist in any and all complex organizations and situations. The next step for the nurse manager is to make a decision to become involved and be willing to learn the rules and "play the game."

Cavanaugh identified five possible categories of strategies to deal with the politics in the health care setting. She terms the use of these strategies by the nurse administrator as "gamesmanship." Cavanaugh's five categories of strategies are as follows[13]:

1. *Disengagement* is the proactive refusal to defend oneself on someone else's terms. It does not suggest that one gives up, but rather that the manager chooses not to pursue the issue further at this particular time.

2. *Offense* is the strategy for taking charge and committing oneself to pursuing a goal at all costs. The nurse manager commits to see the goal through to the end and persists as long as necessary.

3. *Defense* is the strategy to use when one chooses to defend an invasion into his territory. It is a response to an advance by another party.

4. *Building a coalition* is the method of joining forces with another party so that both may obtain goals beyond the reach of each individual. This strategy supports the concept that $1 + 1 = 2$, or the fact that the power that two or more parties create exceeds the sum of their individual power.

5. *Exploiting an opportunity* is using a situation to one's advantage. This does not necessarily mean that an individual takes advantage of another, but rather it is seeing the hidden opportunity in all situations rather than "crying over spilt milk." When a nurse manager views any problem as a potential opportunity to improve or create something better, he/she will be able to create a very positive, productive environment and take advantage of many opportunities overlooked by others. Timing is an essential factor in taking advantage of limited opportunities. The manager must be able and willing to act in a timely manner and be willing to take the associated risks of acting quickly.

Politics may also be defined in terms of social exchange and/ or interaction. Homans (1961) developed the first systematic theory focused on human behavior as an "exchange of activity tangible or intangible, and more or less rewarding or costly between at least two persons."[14] *Social exchange* entails one person or group supplying benefits to another individual or group. This exchange creates future obligations.

Future obligations are a key concept in the politics of an organization. The concept can be a significant source of power for the nurse manager. By assisting a colleague or subordinate attain a goal one has created a *future obligation* that he can collect sometime in the future. When a manager needs a "favor" from a colleague or peer, he or she can "call in the marker" and get the support or assistance needed to accomplish specific goals. This concept is a source of future power for the nurse manager and provides an "invisible" advantage over others.[15] Therefore, a powerful political strategy includes doing things for others to lock in future "invisible" power. It is important, however, that when doing things for others, the nurse manager performs in a sincere, authentic manner. Favors are recognized for what they really are and provide the manager with power only when they are authentic. Sincerity and authenticity are important components of this strategy and can create strong trust relationships. If this trust relationship is nurtured, the bonds of indebtedness and loyalty strengthen. These bonds create, in turn, a unique source of power for both parties in future transactions. This power gives them both a competitive advantage over others. The power obtained from social exchange is a key source of power for the nurse manager to be successful in a political, competitive health care arena.

Politics In the Nonprofit Sector

There are some significant differences between politics in the private and the nonprofit sectors that warrant discussion for the nurse manager. Kennedy's research on nonprofit organizations reveals two inescapable facts about politics in the nonprofit sector.[16]

First, there are actually more politics in a nonprofit organization than in the private sector. Second, employees have a greater chance of being political victims in a nonprofit organization. The research shows that many individuals enter the nonprofit sector or service professions to avoid "cut-throat" politics. These people choose the nonprofit sector to avoid the risks, politics, and "bottom-line" mentality of the business world. The assumption is that individuals trade salary dollars in the nonprofit sector for the security of a nonprofit service organization.

The nonprofit organization conveys the image that the organization is a "service-oriented" family wherein all employees can enjoy paternalistic treatment and strong job security. The irony is, however, that no organization can escape the influence of politics. In the nonprofit organization, politics are merely underground. Wherever groups of individuals with varying perceptions, values, and goals work together, politics exist. Politics are an inescapable part of organizational life in the United States where few homogeneous groups exist.

As the health care industry becomes more overtly competitive, the political process will become more visible and recognized as a normal component of the organization. It is important, therefore, for nurse managers to acknowledge the presence of politics in daily hospital operations and then make the proactive decision to learn how to "play the game." For nurse managers, this can be called the challenge of "learning to play hardball." It is impossible for any health care manager or administrator to be successful without learning this game!

Political Myths and Realities

Before outlining strategies to make the political process work in one's favor, it is necessary to identify a few myths and realities concerning politics in the health care environment. Women generally have not been very eager or enthusiastic about becoming involved in politics in any environment. This trend is changing in the nursing profession. As competition in the health care professions increases and more men enter the profession of nursing, this trend can be expected to change at a faster pace. It is crucial that current and future nursing managers learn differences between the myths and realities of politics so that they can be knowledgeable in this area. Table 9-3 outlines a few of the significant myths and realities of politics.[2]

Developing Political Savvy

After understanding the nature of politics and the impact it has on the organization, it is important for the nurse manager to be able to use the political process to accomplish goals for the nursing department.

Table 9-3   Myths and Realities of Politics

Myths	Realities
1. Hard work and competence always result in success.	1. Success is situational The boss defines what hard work and competence are.
2. Being fired means you are incompetent.	2. There may be no relationship between competence and being fired.
3. Performance appraisals can be objective if done properly.	3. Performance appraisals are always subjective.
4. Office politics is a nasty game, played by bad people.	4. Office politics is a normal organizational process.
5. Individuals are either politically savvy, or they're not.	5. Political savvy is learned.
6. Top management possesses all the political clout.	6. There are some people who are low on the organizational chart, (housekeepers and secretaries) who are actually more powerful than some managers.
7. It is possible to "rise above" the politics in an organization, if you are a responsible, ethical manager.	7. It is impossible not to be involved in politics of the organization if you are performing your job appropriately.

The first strategy a manager can use is the interviewing process and personnel selection to reduce potential conflict situations in a department.[2] A manager must acknowledge that employees they hire could potentially acquire significant political power in the organization that can be used to support or sabotage the manager. Therefore, the value of careful personnel selection cannot be underestimated.

Along the same lines, it is important for managers to set the expectation that employees support them. Nursing administrators have been hesitant to be "up front" and direct with their subordinates regarding their formal support. In many instances, energy, time, and resources have been spent on overcoming overt and covert efforts to undermine and sabotage the nurse manager. A more effective strategy for the nurse manager to use when taking over a new position is to announce to subordinates, "I have earned the right and authority to determine which direction this nursing organization is going. Anyone who is not going in the same direction as I am, or who is unable to support me has a decision to make."

This direct style of communication and leadership allows individuals to know where the manager is coming from and realize what the manager expects from them, as well as the consequences of their actions. When managers try to be too "tactful," employees sometimes do not get the message. A manager never does anyone a favor when he or she avoids dealing with a problem or problem employee. He or she also acquires a reputation of being unable or unwilling to deal with difficult situations. This kind of avoidance behavior usually comes back to haunt the manager. To use an old cliche: Honesty really is the best policy. When managers are honest with their employees, they have a better chance of gaining employee support and respect, and of avoiding political undermining by subordinates.

The political activity that occurs among peers resembles the dynamics of a family. Traditionally, peers in an organization compete with one another, protect one another, squeal on one another, and vie for the attention and favor of the boss. It is important for managers to develop cooperative, supportive, relationships with peers for long-term success. If this cooperation is not present, peers can find many ways to undermine the performance of another. Many good managers have been destroyed by nonsupportive peers. Examples of peer activities that can ruin a manager include the following:

- Feeding the boss questionable "truths" about a manager
- Being resistive, uncooperative, or unavailable in joint projects
- Withholding important information from a peer
- Giving a peer wrong information
- Trying to find fault with a peer. If anyone is looking for errors he will be able to find them because all humans are subject to errors.

A final political arena lies within one's relationship with his boss or superior. The most important political strategy with superiors begins with the "selection" of a boss. The single most important political decision a nurse manager can make lies in the decision of who to work for and when. Many nurses do not even consider this fact as a political issue. When a nurse is considering a new position, the most important factor in that new job is the "fit" with the new superior. The nurse interviewing for a new position should consider this decision critical. It is crucial to select a political arena in which he or she can survive and be successful. Based on individual goals, personalities, and so on, there are some political environments in which specific individuals could not and would not want to survive. The interviewing nurse therefore should select a political environment and boss that "fit" his or her personality.

Other political strategies for the nurse executive/manager to implement to increase one's effectiveness and recognition in the organization include the following:

1. Smiling and cheerfulness are excellent weapons to throw an enemy off guard. This strategy is called the "kill them with kindness" strategy. When a manager is in a very competitive situation with a peer, and each is trying to catch the other one in a mistake, this is a good strategy to throw the competitor off guard. Giving a peer a compliment and being unusually friendly, keeps the peer from knowing what the competition is up to.

2. Identify the credible grapevine and then feed the grapevine information that is important to have circulated. If a hospital is planning smaller merit increases as a result of cost containment pressures, it should anticipate that the staff will be dissatisfied. When it is heard that a nearby hospital is actually laying off nurses because of declining census, it would be politically advantageous to leak that information to the grapevine. When employees hear the rumors, they will realize how bad things are in the entire industry and will be less dissatisfied when they are affected only by the smaller merit increases. It is important always to be honest in the information that is passed to the grapevine. If false information is passed on, the manager's credibility will be questioned forever.

   The grapevine is also very useful to test the organizational climate at a specific point in time. The grapevine will let the manager know if the staff is uneasy or generally optimistic. The nurse manager can then plan to time strategies and programs based on the hospital's "mental" health at any one time.

   When and if the grapevine is essentially quiet and nothing is going on, the manager should feed it some positive information that he wants circulated. The grapevine cannot tolerate "no news," and so if nothing is actually happening, people will make up information to fill the vacuum. This could be potentially destructive to individuals or the organization as a whole.

3. If the manager has a flexible work schedule, it is actually better to work late in the evening than come in early.[2] When one works later than boss or peers, there are more witnesses to his or her devotion. When a manager is the first to arrive in the morning, there are few people there to

witness the manager's loyalty to the job. Exhibiting devotion and dedication to one's job is a political plus from a boss' perspective. On the other hand, that same dedication and devotion can create feelings of resentment and jealousy from peers. This particular strategy can be a two-edged sword, and only the manager can determine which consequences he is most comfortable dealing with.

4. A manager should always read what the boss reads. The author learned this political tactic from her secretary, Beverly. By reading what the boss reads, the manager has a sneak preview of what the boss is thinking and believes is important. One can anticipate future strategies placing him in a position to respond in a proactive and timely manner to the boss' requests.

5. Another key strategy is to actively listen to one's secretary. Secretaries are some of the most powerful individuals in the organization. They have access to privileged information, conversations, and intuitive feelings. They are the advocates and protectors of the nurse manager in the "political underground" of the organization. A savvy nurse manager should listen very closely to the observations and suggestions of his or her secretary. It is a smart political strategy never to underestimate the power and perceptiveness of one's secretary or other administrative secretaries in the organization.

An ideal political strategy to increase one's prestige and image as a nurse manager could be to hire a male secretary.[2] If the nurse executive is a woman, a male secretary could magnify the prestige of the nurse executive. When male executives speak to a male secretary they experience a subconscious fear that they could end up in such a subordinate role, and they are put off guard.

No matter what sex a secretary is, there is nothing that will assist a manager's political position more than a perceptive, loyal, trustworthy secretary. It is impossible for any one individual to be on top of all the political activities occurring in an organization. A good secretary is a strong asset in furthering one's career, and can keep the manager on top of issues on an ongoing basis. Key political responsibilities for an executive secretary include the following:

- Always make the nurse manager look good.
- Supply the nurse manager with key information from other executive secretaries and grapevine sources.
- Maintain documentation of all key issues to support the executive.

- Remind the manager of personal dates, courtesies, birthdates, etc.
- Screen individuals who seek access to the manager.
- Alert the nurse manager of trouble that is brewing in any department or with any other managers.

The overall importance of a sharp, loyal secretary cannot be overemphasized for the successful political survival of the nurse manager.

6. Make the decision that learning "the rules of the game" to obtain a goal is more important than being right. Historically this has been very difficult for some nurse managers to work through in their minds. Nurses tend to be focused on the issue of being right and being able to gain recognition for being right. In a political environment, many times one needs to sacrifice being "right" on an issue for the sake of "winning the war" or obtaining the goal.

   For example, nurse managers get very frustrated with angry, aggressive, demanding physician behavior. Frequently they want to deal with this behavior by confrontation. The political reality in a hospital is that if there is an outright confrontation between a nurse and a physician, the physician possesses more legitimate power and will always win in the long run. The nurse may win the issue, but because the medical staff has more aggregate power than the nursing staff, they will be able to win the long-term battle through methods such as refusing to support nursing programs and sabotage. It is crucial for nurse managers to acknowledge that physicians have significant political power in the hospital and attempt to make all confrontations with them win–win situations.

7. Negotiation strategies are important tools in the political arena of a hospital. Negotiation is a cooperative strategy whereby participants are persuaded to strive for goals that are of value to all who participate. The use of negotiation in political situations means there is a greater possibility for each of the participants to reach successful cooperative goals.[17]

   Negotiation requires a process of give-and-take to reach a win–win situation for all parties. This goal of win–win by definition eliminates the possibility of one party being right and the other one being wrong. This is a significant issue for many nurse managers. The way to overcome this mental hurdle is for the nurse manager to rephrase his or her goals. An example of a rephrased goal for a nurse manager could include

- *Goal:* Make sure one has accurate and complete information so that he or she may eliminate errors and reduce conflict situations with physicians.
- *Rephrased Goal:* Assist the physician to attain his goals so that he may support the manager in obtaining his or her goals.

The manager may operate in a very forthright, honest, and ethical manner to obtain this latter goal. It is smart to assist others in obtaining their goals as a strategy to obtain individual goals. This is a cardinal principle in establishing political savvy in the organization, so that the manager can attain the goals the organization expects him to accomplish.

There are a few famous quotes by successful individuals that portray this principal very graphically.

> You can get anything in life you want, if you help enough other people get what they want.
> Zig Ziglar

> It is one of the most beautiful compensations in life, that no man can sincerely try to help another, without helping himself.
> Ralph Waldo Emerson

Additional strategies to acquire political savvy to maximize one's opportunities in the organization include the following[15]:

- Identify the powerful people in the organization and align oneself with them.
- Socialize with powerful people.
- Work hard and volunteer for extra projects and responsibilities.
- Know who the competition and/or enemy is.
- Do not take unnecessary risks but be aggressive and visible.
- Know the job, the company, and the business.
- Develop excellent communication skills.
- Know the boss and his preferences and "hot buttons."

INCREASING PERSONAL POWER

It has already been established that a manager requires personal power to be effective in accomplishing personal and organizational goals. This personal power cannot be obtained overnight, and so an individual should "fake it, until he can make it." This means that nurse managers should "act as if" they have the personal power required to accomplish their goals until they actually do have the power.

In order to "act as if" one has power, one must be aware of how a powerful person acts and looks. The look and acting requires an awareness of the message they communicate and a decision by the manager to develop and practice them on an ongoing basis.

The perception of others that one possesses power actually increases one's personal power. Perceptions are reality to the person who has the perceptions, whether they are accurate perceptions or not. Therefore, if a manager can create the illusion of being powerful to other people, they treat him "as if" he really is powerful. Thus, a beginning strategy for developing personal power is to "act as if" one is really powerful. This strategy creates the illusion that the manager has personal power by assuming the traits, behaviors, and characteristics that society and other people interpret as being associated with power. By deciding to incorporate the traits, looks, and characteristics of power that one feels comfortable with into one's professional image, the nurse manager will be perceived by others as possessing personal power.

Table 9-4 outlines various characteristics, looks, and symbols that society perceives as being associated with personal power. The nurse manager could incorporate any of these characteristics into his or her image as a strategy to increase personal power.

Management training programs are beginning to incorporate executive behavior skills into their curricula. Debra Benson teaches "boss behavior" in her "Executive Presence" Workshop to create the illusion of power for the executive. An example of such "boss behavior" includes the strategy of pausing at the door for a few seconds before entering a room to establish one's presence.[18]

A nurse manager can best acquire charismatic or referent power by developing a well-defined goal or vision for excellence. The goal or vision generates support from subordinates, giving the nurse manager power or influence over them. Others

Table 9-4 Looks and Characteristics of Power

Characteristic	Interpretation
Assertive, confident gait	The person has specific goals, and possesses the knowledge, expertise, and power to accomplish those goals.
A healthy, physically fit look	The individual is in control of his physical body, and therefore must also be able to control other areas. He or she also probably possesses the stamina required to lead under difficult situations.
A strong, confident handshake	The person is direct, is trustworthy, is in control, and has a strong ego.
Good, upright posture	The person belongs, is confident, and knows what's happening.
High visibility	The person is very powerful, hard working, and successful.
Good eye contact	The person is direct, is trustworthy, and has nothing to hide.

are attracted to the manager because of his or her strong vision of the future and strong commitment to attain the visionary goal. Individuals respond to leaders who can lead them toward exceptional goals and accomplishments. They are inspired by leaders who can make things happen and desire to be a part of such a phenomenon. They follow willingly just to be a part of the excitement and do not require any visible rewards or threats of punishments.

It is important for the nurse to identify the ideal model of power, including the ideal way a manager should look and act. By imagining oneself as already possessing personal power and performing in powerful ways, the manager provides the subconscious mind with an ideal model of how one should perform. This ideal model can replace old, nonpowerful behaviors that existed in one's past. Visualization of the ideal self is a method of rehearsal that results in perfect practice. Only perfect practice leads to perfect performance.

The main goal in visualization is to imagine or see in one's mind the ideal way an individual wishes to look and behave, given specific goals. This ideal behavior includes how one looks, what one says, and how one responds to others. The visualization of the ideal self must include a recipe for these various aspects of one's professional image. Daily visualization will alter one's present subconscious image of self, which is really like reprogramming the software of one's mind.[19]

Schwartz advocates a little different strategy for acquiring power in his book, *The Magic of Getting What You Want*.[20] His strategy is called the *ASK method* and dictates that one ASKS for what is wanted or needed. This method actually originated in the Bible with the phrase, "Ask and it shall be given unto you, Seek and ye shall find, Knock and it shall be opened unto you."

There is real power in asking directly for the specific things one desires. Examples for the nurse manager include the following:

- Ask successful people for their advice.
- Ask for a promotion.
- Ask people, don't order them around.

Another strategy for accumulating personal power is through practice or role playing. Role playing provides insight into another person's thoughts, feelings, and motivations, so that the manager can plan the most effective strategy to accomplish his goals. When one anticipates another's responses or reactions, it is possible to develop the strategy that minimizes resistance and maximizes support toward the goal.

In 1957 the American Management Association was the first to use role playing as a method of executive development.[20] Adopting such role playing or acting skills does not mean becoming a fake. Rather, it assists in learning how to communicate better with authority, confidence, energy, and responsiveness.

This is a very good strategy for nurse managers to utilize when they need to terminate an employee, confront a peer or physician, or ask for a raise. Any difficult situation can go more smoothly if the manager has practiced or role played the situation before the actual encounter. By role playing the situation in his or her mind with a trusted colleague, the leader can anticipate potential responses or reactions of the other party and build self-confidence by being prepared.

Self-confidence is a very important by-product of being prepared. Being prepared is, in turn, a by-product of practice or rehearsing what to say and how to say it in a controlled, relaxed environment. If one practices using a tape recorder and/or mirror, one can get a good idea of how one comes across. A trusted colleague can also provide the feedback needed to improve.

When rehearsing for such encounters, it must be remembered that eye contact is a very powerful component of one's image. The simple act of looking someone squarely in the eye is more persuasive than a hundred words.[22] Eye contact mandates a response and communicates that the manager is direct, is trustworthy, and is not hiding anything.

Authenticity is a characteristic that requires attention throughout a discussion of personal power. Authenticity is a powerful strategy and is more important than being accurate or perfect. Authenticity is being real or true to oneself. Authenticity is making changes but not taking on any characteristics that make one feel uncomfortable or of which one disapproves. Authenticity is wearing clothes that make one comfortable. Authenticity is adopting only characteristics that "fit" with one's personality. Subordinates admire leaders who can acknowledge their own "humanness," rather than attempting to appear perfect, superior, or always in control. Being authentic involves the risk of being seen as a mortal being capable of making mistakes, and admitting those mistakes. The truly confident leader is willing to show his human side, without fear of damaging his overall image.

Power Looks, Habits, Symbols, and Dress

Personal image and appearance are very important in communicating self-confidence and the ability to accomplish goals. People make assumptions about an individual based on the way the person looks and dresses.

In the business world, there are very specific messages that are communicated by clothes and accessories. The suit has long been associated as a symbol of power and authority. On the other hand, the white uniform of the nurse has long been associated with a "subordinate" role. The nurse executive or manager makes a bold statement when trading in her white uniform for a business suit.

Within a very short period of time the nurse manager realizes that he or she receives more respect from physicians, staff, and other departments by replacing the white uniform with a suit or other type of street clothes. By dressing as an executive staff member, he or she commands more respect and credibility without actually changing anything else.

Because 95% of all nurse managers and executives are female, the author will focus on the specific aspects and implications of dress for the female. These ideas about dress and accessories have been obtained from observation and speculation. They have no scientific origin but are unwritten "rules" in the business world. The ideas are learned through observation of role models or mentors. It is not written anywhere that a nurse manager or executive must do any of these things. However, these factors have been observed to contribute to the image and illusion of power for those who have incorporated the concepts into their professional and personal image.

Suits communicate a more confident, powerful image than do dresses. Dresses, however, can be very appropriate and a pleasant change of pace from wearing suits on a daily basis. However, if dresses are worn, frills, ruffles, low-cut necklines, and see-through material should be avoided. These fashions communicate that the nurse manager is more a female than a manager, and this is not the message one wants to communicate at work.

Along the same lines, plain leather pumps are more business-like than fancy shoes with open toes, buttons, or bows. The latter features emphasize the fact that the manager is a woman. There is nothing wrong with being a woman, but extremely feminine clothes and accessories are best confined to social occasions, rather than being worn in the workplace.

Colors communicate various messages and set the tone for interpersonal encounters. The navy blue suit is considered the most powerful of all wardrobes. In many circles, executives actually talk about wearing their blue "power" suit when they anticipate a difficult meeting or encounter.

Gray communicates diplomacy, whereas black is considered a very authoritative color. Red is viewed as either aggressive or frightening. When one wears a red outfit, people tend to focus on the wardrobe rather than on what is being said. Therefore, red can be very distracting. Beige or tan communicates a neutral or open position and is very nonthreatening. Brown, on the other hand, communicates a depressed mood. Mauve or purple, which is a combination of blue and red communicates power with a hint of aggression. Yellow communicates a certain frivolity and should not be worn in a confrontation or power situation if one wants to be taken seriously. White communicates a sense of space and freedom, whereas pink is a very calming color that can be worn to diffuse aggressive feelings or actions.

The interpretation of the meanings and implications of these colors is far from being scientific. The implications have been identified by simple observation and supposition. If the nurse manager truly wants to maximize her chances of success and the establishment of an adequate power base, it is a good idea to leave nothing to chance. These helpful hints have proved to be beneficial to successful leaders in their career development.

On the opposite side of the coin, there are some specific behaviors and/or habits that are important to avoid in one's development of power and authority. These habits communicate a lack of self-confidence and power, whether that is true or not. Some of these habits are shown in Table 9-5.

A fair amount of time has been spent discussing various aspects of clothing, image, looks, and habits that contribute to one's perceived power base. This approach may seem somewhat superficial because of its focus on creating the illusion of power. It is important to mention that these image-building strategies should supplement the acquisition of expert knowledge and charisma. Expert knowledge is obtained through continued academic achievements, involvement with a mentor, and expe-

Table 9-5 Habits To Be Avoided

Habit	Message Communicated
1. Licking lips Sweating Nail biting Fidgeting Tapping fingers or feet	Person is nervous and unsure of himself.
2. Poor posture	Individual lacks self-confidence and goal direction.
3. Blinking or excessive eye movements	Individual has something to hide, is shifty. Individual has poor self-image.
4. Wrinkled clothes	Individual has poor self-image.

rience. Charismatic characteristics are developed through a commitment to personal introspection and growth. The truly motivated nurse manager or executive will benefit by using the combination of strategies that best fits his/her personality and professional goals.

SUMMARY

This chapter has discussed the role and importance of power and politics for the nurse manager or executive in a competitive health care environment. Some of the most salient concepts presented include the following:

1. *Authority* is the legitimate power granted an individual by the organization as a result of his or her position.

2. *Referent* and *expert power* are earned by the individual by acquiring knowledge and charisma. Employees willingly follow leaders with referent or expert power because they respect their opinions and ideas.

3. The effective nurse manager needs to acquire both legitimate and earned power to maintain a balanced power base and the respect of staff.

4. The *political process* is an inevitable component of management in organizations because individuals have varying goals and objectives, and resources are limited.

5. *Power* is a neutral force that allows a manager to accomplish personal, organizational, and professional goals.

6. Janet Hagberg outlined six stages of power through which leaders progress in their leadership development:

   Stage One: The Dictators
   Stage Two: The Seducers
   Stage Three: The Great Persuaders
   Stage Four: The Role Models
   Stage Five: The Empowerers
   Stage Six: The Sages

7. The political "game" includes four basic concepts: the players; the goals, interests, and stakes of the players; the amount of power each player has; and the rules and rewards of the game.

8. There are actually more politics in a nonprofit organization than in a private organization. The politics are merely underground.

9. The development of good interpersonal relationships is the

most effective management strategy to deal with organizational politics.

10. Executive secretaries are very powerful individuals in the organization and can make a significant contribution to a nurse manager's career.

11. It is important for nurse managers to make the decision to learn the "rules of the politics game" and then play to win!

REFERENCES

1. Friss LO: Work force policy perspectives: Registered Nurse. J Health, Policy, Law 5(4) Winter 1981
2. Korda M: , Power! How to Get It, How to Use It. New York, Ballentine Books, 1975
3. Szilagyi A Jr, Wallace M Jr: Organizational Behavior and Performance. Santa Monica, CA, Goodyear Publishing Company, Inc, 1980
4. Hagberg JO: Real Power. Minneapolis, Winston Press, 1984
5. Blau P: Interaction: Social exchange. Encyclopedia of Social Sciences, pp 425-457
6. Clarke JR: Executive Power. Englewood Cliffs, NJ, Prentice Hall, 1979
7. Eisen J: Powertalk. New York, Cornerstone Library, 1984
8. Blau P: Exchange and Power in Social Life. New York, John Wiley & Sons, 1964
9. Katz D, Kahn R: The Social Psychology of Organizations, p 528. New York, John Wiley & Sons, 1966
10. Hagberg JO: The good, the bad, the ugly. Savvy October 1984
11. Allison GT: Essence of Decision, p 144. Boston, Little, Brown & Co, 1971
13. Cavanaugh D: Gamesmanship: The art of strategizing. JONA p 39, April 1985
14. Homans G: Social Behavior: Its Elementary Forms. New York, Hartcourt Press, 1961
15. Posner M: Executive Essentials, p 266. New York, Avon Books, 1982
16. Kennedy MM: Office Politics. New York, Warner Books, 1980
17. Nierenberg G: The Art of Negotiating, p 25. New York, Cornerstone Library, 1968
18. Vogel M: That quality of charisma: Projecting your special something. Human Potential p 13, May 1985
19. Goldberg P: Rehearsing for risk: Practice makes possible. Human Potential p 30, May 1985
20. Schwartz DJ: The Magic of Getting What You Want, p 159. New York, William Morrow & Co, 1983
21. Geltner S: Learning to play the part. Human Potential p 19, May 1985
22. Carr A: Business as a Game. New York, A Mentor Book, New American Library, 1968

ADDITIONAL READINGS

1. Girard J: How to Sell Yourself. New York, Warner Books, 1981
2. Harragan BL: Games Mother Never Taught You: Corporate Gamesmanship for Women. New York, Warner Books, 1977
3. Gabarro J: When a new manager takes charge. Harvard Business Rev May-June 1985
4. Kennedy MM: Powerbase: How to Build It, How to Keep It. New York, Macmillan, 1984
5. Leminger M: The leadership crisis in nursing. JONA 4(2):28-34, 1974
6. Malloy JT: Malloy's Live for Success. New York, Morrow, 1981
7. Malloy JT: The Woman's Dress for Success Book. New York, Warner Books, 1977
8. Peterson GG: Power: A perspective for the nurse administrator. JONA 9(7):7-10

Glossary

Accelerated method of depreciation: The method that charges off more of the original cost of the fixed asset in the earlier years than in the later years of the asset's service life.

Accounts receivable: An amount that is owed to the business by one of its customers, as a result of the ordinary extension of credit.

Accounting period: The period of time over which an income statement summarizes the changes in owners' equity, usually 1 year.

Accrual basis of accounting: The recording of revenues and expenses as they occur, irrespective of when revenue is received or expenses are paid.

Accumulated depreciation: An account showing the total amount of depreciation of an asset that has been accumulated to date.

Acid-test ratio: The ratio obtained by dividing current assets by current liabilities.

Admitting diagnosis: The condition that best describes on admission why the patient is being admitted to the hospital.

Allocated cost: The apportionment of indirect overhead expenses that get distributed to patient care departments in a full cost-accounting system.

Amortization: The process of writing off the cost of intangible assets.

Asset: An item which is owned by the business that has value and can be measured objectively.

Auditing: A review of accounting records by independent, outside public accountants.

Authority: The legitimate right to require compliance from subordinates on the basis of position.

Bad debts: The amount of credit sales that will never be collected.

Balance sheet: A financial statement that reports the assets and liabilities of a company at one point in time. Assets are listed on the left and liabilities on the right.

Bond: A written promise to repay money furnished the business with interest at some future date, usually 5 or more years in the future.

Capital stock: A balance account showing the amount that was assigned to the shares of stock at the time they were originally issued.

Case mix index: The factor that identifies the complexity of the cases treated or services delivered by a health care institution.

Cash basis accounting: An accounting system that records transactions when cash is actually received or paid out.

Common stock: Stock whose owners are not entitled to preferential treatment with regard to dividends or to the distribution of assets in the event of liquidation.

Consolidated statements: Financial statements prepared for a corporate family as one entity.

Consumption: The purchasing of goods or services for the use of the individual.

Contribution margin: The excess of gross revenue over direct costs.

Cost accounting: The process of identifying total costs and assigning them to the service that the company produces.

Cost of goods sold: The cost of the merchandise sold to the consumer.

Cost per case: The expense to a hospital to care for a specific patient from admission to discharge.

Credit: The right-hand side of an account or an amount entered on the right-hand side of an account.

Creditor: A person who lends money or extends credit to a business.

Current assets: Assets which are either currently in the form of cash or are expected to be converted into cash within a short period of time, usually 1 year.

Current liabilities: Obligations that become due within a short period of time, usually 1 year.

Current ratio: The ratio obtained by dividing the total current assets by the total of the current liabilities.

Curriculum vitae: A resume that is designed for the purpose of presenting educational and experiential qualifications of a professional.

Days in receivables: The number of days of sales that are tied up in accounts receivable.

Debit: The left-hand side of an account or an amount entered on the left-hand side of an account.

Debt capital: The capital raised by the issuance of bonds.

Debt ratio: The ratio obtained by dividing debt capital by total capital.

Deferred revenue: A liability that arises when a customer pays a business in advance for a service or product. It is liability because the business has no obligation to render the service.

Delphi method: A group-decision technique closely associated with the nominal group process.

Demand: A schedule of alternative quantities of a good or service that a person or group of people is willing to purchase at alternative prices during a specified period of time.

Depreciation: The process of recognizing a portion of the cost of an asset as an expense during each year of its estimated service life.

Depreciation rate: The percentage of the cost of an asset that is charged off each year.

Dividend: The funds generated by profitable operations that are distributed to the shareholders.

Double-declining balance method: An accelerated method of depreciation.

Earnings: Another term for income.

Earnings per share: A ratio obtained by dividing the total earnings for a given period of time by the number of shares of common stock outstanding.

Elasticity: The measure of response to changes in quantity demanded relative to changes in prices.

Equity: Claims against assets that are held by owners or by creditors of a corporation.

Equity capital: The capital raised from the resources owned by the corporation.

Estimated net cost: The difference between the cost of a fixed asset and its estimated residual value.

Estimated tax liability: The amount estimated to be owed to the government for taxes.

Expenditure: A liability arising from the acquisition of an asset.

Expense: A decrease in owners' equity resulting from operations.

Expensing: The process of charging the cost of an asset to the company as an expense.

Expert power: The capacity to influence based on some skill, expertise, or knowledge.

Face amount: The total amount of a loan, specified on the face of bond that must be repaid.

FIFO: The inventory method that assumes that the goods that enter the inventory first are the first to be sold.

Fixed assets: The tangible properties with relatively long life span, generally used in the production of goods and services rather than being held for resale.

Good will: An intangible asset; an amount paid for a favorable location or reputation.

Gross margin: The difference between sales revenue and cost of goods sold.

Grapevine: A slang term referring to informal communication networks within the organization.

Horizontal integration: A company seeks ownership control of some of its competitors.

Inflation: The erosion of real income by price increases. Inflation places pressures on organizational fiscal-reward policies.

Income statement: A statement of revenues and expenses for a given period; a flow report.

Indirect overhead: Costs that cannot be identified with specific services rendered by patient care departments or patient support departments and that therefore is allocated to departments on a reasonable basis.

Inventories: Goods being held for sale, and material and partially finished products that will be sold upon completion.

Inventory turnover: Tells how many items of inventory were totally replaced during the year; calculated by dividing the average inventory into cost of goods sold.

Investments: Securities that are held for a relatively long period of time and are purchased for reasons other than the temporary use of excess cash. They are not current assets.

Lease: An agreement under which the owner of property permits someone else to use it.

Ledger: A group of accounts.

Liability: The equity or claim of a creditor.

LIFO: The last-in, first-out inventory method, which assumes that the last goods purchased are the first to be sold.

Liquid assets: Cash and assets which are easily converted into cash.

Liquidity ratios: The relationship of obligations coming due to assets that should provide the cash for meeting these obligations.

Loss-leader pricing: A popular product or service is priced low to attract a large number of buyers who are also expected to buy other products.

Marginal costing: The assignment of only marginal or variable costs to an activity or department as contrasted with full costing.

Market: A market is the set of all actual and potential buyers of a product.

Marketing: A human activity directed at satisfying needs and wants through the exchange process.

Marketing mix: A set of controllable variables and their levels that the firm uses to influence the target market.

Marketing strategy: Set of objectives, policies, and rules that determine the firm's marketing efforts over time.

Market value: The amount for which an asset can be sold in the marketplace.

Marketable securities: Securities that are expected to be converted into cash within a year; a current asset.

Matching concept: Costs are matched against the revenue of a period.

Mentor: A trusted counselor or guide who assists a professional attain career goals.

Mortgage: A pledge of real estate as security for a loan.

Negotiate: The process of two parties coming together to discuss, debate, and compromise.

Net book value: The difference between the cost of a fixed asset and its accumulated depreciation.

Net income: The amount by which total revenues exceed total expenses for a given period.

Net loss: The amount by which total expenses exceed total revenues for a given period.

Network: A system of interconnected or cooperated individuals.

Note receivable: An amount that is evidenced by a promissory note.

Obsolescence: A loss in the usefulness of an asset because of the development of improved equipment, changes in style, or other causes not related to the physical condition of the asset.

Operating expenses: Costs associated with sales and administrative activities as distinct from those associated with product of goods or services.

Overhead: Any cost of doing business other than a direct cost of a service.

Owner's equity: The claims of owners against the assets of a business.

Par value: The specific amount printed on the face of a stock certificate.

Physical inventory: The counting of all merchandise currently on hand.

Power: The ability to accomplish one's goals.

Preferred stock: Its owners receive preferential treatment with regard to dividends or with regard to the distribution of assets in the event of liquidation.

Prepaid expenses: Services and certain intangibles purchased prior to the period during which their benefits are received; treated as assets until they are consumed.

Price-earnings ratio: A ratio obtained by dividing the average market price of the stock by the earnings per share.

Profit margin: Net income expressed as a percentage of net sales.

Per diem reimbursement: A flat per day reimbursement rate irrespective of the services delivered to the patient that day.

Price: The ratio of exchange between two commodities.

Pricing strategy: The task of determining the price range and price movement through time that supports the company's sales and profit objectives.

Primary diagnosis: The condition that best describes the services the patient actually receives during hospitalization.

Principal diagnosis: The condition that best describes, after study, why a patient needed to be admitted to the hospital.

Product life cycle: The attempt to recognize distinct stages in the sales history of a product or service (introduction, growth, maturity, decline).

Product line management: Managing a hospital's services by product line based on profit or loss potential.

Prospective reimbursement: Reimbursement or payment schedules are set or determined before the services are delivered.

Quick assets: Current assets other than inventory and prepaid expenses.

Referent power: The capacity to influence based on an individual's identification with an impressive individual.

Retained earnings: The increase in the shareholders' equity as a result of profitable company operations.

Retrospective reimbursement: Reimbursement or payment for services after they are delivered or received.

Return: The amount earned on invested funds during a period.

Return on shareholders' investment: A ratio obtained by dividing the return by the average amount of shareholders' investment for a period.

Revenue: An increase in owners' equity resulting from operations.

Security: An instrument such as a stock or bond.

Service life: The period of time over which an asset is estimated to be of service to the company.

Shareholders: The owners of an incorporated business.

Solvency: The ability to meet long-term obligations.

Statement of changes in financial position: A financial statement explaining the changes that have occurred in assets, liability, and owners' equity items in an accounting period.

Stock dividend: A dividend consisting of shares of stock in the corporation.

Straightline method: A depreciation method that charges off an equal fraction of the cost of a fixed asset over each year of its service life.

Strategic management process: The managerial process of developing and maintaining a viable relationship between the organization and its environment by developing a mission, goals, strategies, and operational plans.

Supply: The quantity of a good or service present in the marketplace for consumers to purchase.

Target market: The specific market or population that a company seeks to sell to.

Taxable income: The amount of income subject to income tax, computed according to the rules of the Internal Revenue Service.

Transaction: A business event that is recorded in the accounting records.

Transferred cost: The passage of the costs of goods and services from some departments to the user departments.

Trim points: The low and high days for length of stay for each DRG. If a case is within these trim points, the health care institution will get reimbursed a flat per discharge rate irrespective of the specific services delivered to the patient.

Utility: The term used to define the value of a good or service to an individual or society.

Utility function: The perception of the consumer regarding the value of a product or service.

Wage index: The factor that compares wages paid in health care institutions across the nation.

Index